THE HEALING POWER OF ENZYMES

Dear Kerri,
my best + love,
DicQie

DicQie Fuller-Looney,
Ph.D., Dr. Sc., ND, CNC

The Healing Power of Enzymes: Revised Edition

Preface

I first began *The Healing Power of Enzymes* in 1990 after receiving letters from an agent at Prentice Hall requesting that I write a book. At first I was very confused why they asked me to become an author since I did not feel I could do a book justice. Evidently they knew about my clinical research involving typing people into four groups, establishing their differences, and treating them with nutrition and supplemental digestive enzymes. I continued to ignore the persistent agent because I was very busy in my clinic, plus I created a corporation supplying doctors with my clinical formulations called "Transformation Enzymes."

After moving to Scottsdale in 1992 to give myself time to refresh my research and my thought processes, I began to think about how I could begin the book. I got back to the agent and much to my amazement found he was still interested. I had a talk radio show at that time, in which I answered questions about enzyme therapy and nutrition. Based on listeners' questions and how they responded to my answers, I recognized I was actually identifying their type over the air. Once again the book was put to the side as I pursued this new dimension along with the growth of my traveling and teaching. That is until 1994 while speaking at a seminar I met my husband Ken. He came up front as a volunteer to be typed and then arranged for me to come through Houston on a speaking engagement.

The rest is history, and I eventually moved everything I owned, along with my children and my company, to Texas. My husband is a businessman, and while helping build the business, he suggested I get back to the book. By now it was 1995 and I was sure they wrote me off and would not even know who I was if

I phoned. I wrote a letter assuming it would be declined but instead received a phone call and we were back on! The good news is I actually finished the first rendition of this book but the surprise after all those years was the agent wanted me to write about food enzymes rather than supplemental enzymes. It was believed back then that we could actually utilize the enzymes in raw fruits and vegetables. Problem was that by 1995, research had been done to prove that these food enzymes became dormant and unusable in the digestive tract of a human. We agreed to not agree, but they were kind and let me keep my intellectual property rights and up-front money.

The long awaited book was finished, the type and cover agreed upon but no publisher. Within a week, a visitor from Forbes Publishing offered to publish the book. This is the third rewrite and the reason is the world of nutritional science is ever-changing. Forbes closed down their book section since then but maintains their magazine division.

NEW UPDATED INFORMATION AND ADDITIONAL CHAPTERS

The purpose of *The Healing Power of Enzymes* is to give a simple yet comprehensive explanation of enzymes starting from metabolic enzymes (those you produce), when they are produced, and how or when they are turned on or off by one's own DNA.

Something not done before in a book—I include enzyme labeling, a chart of the various supplemental enzymes, what they are produced from, and what foods they break down. It is pertinent information whether you are a first-time reader or a practitioner in Enzyme Therapy. Measurements of enzymes are also attended to since there is a great deal of confusion.

The Internet has brought to the forefront a great deal of information along with nutritional myths and dubious recommendations. I address many of these concerns using my clinical and scientific background. Most chapters will have detailed information on conditions and suggestions on the choices to bring you once again into the best balance you are equipped to maintain. Chapters will either have case studies, testimonials, or both.

RECOGNIZE AND LEARN ABOUT YOUR OWN BIOCHEMICAL TYPE

Because we are all so diverse, you will learn of your own Biochemical Type with one's own specific requirements and enzyme needs. Each Biochemical Type will have defined information and guidance from foods, nutrients, enzyme supplementation, and exercise. The list of foods for each type will either bring balance to your system or will cause inflammatory problems and toxicity issues.

Foods that we are unable to properly break down will ferment, turn rancid, or putrefy in our system.

EVERYTHING YOU KNEW ABOUT CALORIES IS WRONG

You will not see references made to calorie-counting in this book. The only time a calorie may be mentioned is when making a point. I earned a PhD in Dietetic Nutrition and the theory about calorie calculation has bothered me for more years than I want to mention. Food is energy for the body. Digestive enzymes in the mouth, stomach, and intestines break up complex food molecules into simpler structures, such as sugars and amino acids that travel through the bloodstream to all our tissues. Our cells use the energy stored in the chemical bonds of these simpler molecules to carry on business as usual. This is a simplistic statement about nutrition based on perfect conditions. If only we were perfect.

I was taught a scientific theory on calorie calculation based on American chemist Wilbur Olin Atwater from the 19th century. The available energy in all foods was calculated with a unit known as the food calorie, or kilocalorie—the amount of energy required to heat one kilogram of water by one degree Celsius. Fats provide approximately nine calories per gram, whereas carbohydrates and proteins deliver just four. Fiber offers a piddling two calories because enzymes in the human digestive tract have great difficulty breaking it up into smaller molecules. Atwater was doing his best, but no food is average. Each food source we eat is digested or unable to be digested in its own way.

According to Rob Dunn, a biologist at North Carolina State University, new research has revealed that this assumption is, at best, far too simplistic. To accurately calculate the total calories that someone gets out of a given food, you would have to take into account a dizzying array of factors, including whether that food has evolved to survive digestion; how boiling, baking, microwaving, genetically modifying it, or barbecuing it changes its structure and chemistry; how much energy the body expends to break down different kinds of food; and the extent to which the billions of bacteria in the gut aid human digestion and, conversely, steal some calories for themselves.

Nutrition scientists are beginning to learn enough to hypothetically improve calorie labels, but digestion turns out to be such a fantastically complex and messy affair that we will probably never derive a formula for an infallible calorie count. Rachel N. Carmody working in research states: *"Even if two people eat the same sweet potato or piece of meat cooked the same way, they will not get the same number of calories out of it."*

People also vary in the particular enzymes they produce or genetically turned on by their own DNA. By some measures, most adults do not produce the enzyme lactase, which is necessary to break down lactose sugars in milk. As a result, one man's high-calorie latte is another's low-calorie case of the diarrhea.

People differ immensely as well in what scientists have come to regard as an extra organ of the human body—the community of bacteria living in the intestines. Because the extra bacteria make them more efficient at metabolizing food: so instead of being lost as waste, more nutrients make their way into the circulation and, if they go unused, get stored as fat.

Many modern diets contain so many easily digestible processed foods; they may be reducing the populations of gut microbes that evolved to digest the more fibrous matter our own enzymes cannot. If we continue to make our gut a less friendly environment for such bacteria, we may get fewer calories (energy) from tough foods such as celery.

Even if we entirely revamped calorie counts, however, they would never be precisely accurate because the amount of calories we extract from food depends on such a complex interaction between food and each human body and its many personalized microbes.

WHY CALORIE MATH DOESN'T WORK FOR WEIGHT LOSS

A calorie is not a calorie when you eat it at a different time of day.

A calorie is not a calorie when you eat it in a different processed form.

A calorie is not a calorie if two people eating the same food utilize it differently.

Always eat carbohydrate calories in a very calculated way.

The more you exercise, the more your body will tolerate carbohydrates.

Most people will burn fat faster when restricting fat?

ARE ANY OF THE ABOVE STATEMENTS TRUE?

Biochemical Scientists do not accept the measurement of calories. In fact, they do not believe you can truly measure calories based on so many different and diverse reasonings. Many of these reasons have to do with the energy expenditure of the foods themselves—how they were grown, prepared, and who eats them.

People vary in the particular digestive enzymes they produce.

> **Some people produce more proteases for digesting proteins, others lipases for fat breakdown, and carbohydrate-splitting enzymes for digesting carbohydrates.**
>
> **Digestive enzyme production is as different as fingerprints because it is based on their own DNA.**
>
> **People differ immensely as the bacteria that live within them.**
>
> **Extra or diverse bacteria make them more efficient at metabolizing food: so instead of being lost as waste, more nutrients make their way into the circulation, or if they go unused, get stored as fat.**
>
> **Calorie math will never be precisely accurate because the amount of calories we extract from food depends on such a complex interaction between food and each human body with its many microbes.**

I believe the summation is correct and have spent more than the last 30 years trying to make sense out of all of it. Dr. Rogers J. Williams first coined the phrase, "Biochemical Individualism" back in the 1960s while working at the University of Texas. I grabbed onto his theory because it made so much sense to me and have been diligently making it a science ever since.

I want to introduce you to another scientist who has dedicated a great deal of his life to understanding calories and weight gain. Gary Taubes, co-founder of the Nutrition Science Initiative and author of *Why We Get Fat: And What to Do about It*, asks:

> *Why do so many of us get so fat? The answer appears obvious. "The fundamental cause of obesity and overweight," the World Health Organization says, "is an energy imbalance between calories consumed and calories expended." Put simply, we either eat too much or are too sedentary, or both. By this logic, any excess of calories—whether from protein, carbohydrate, or fat (the three main components, or "macro-nutrients," in food)—will inevitably pack on the pounds.*

He goes on to question the theory we have been brought up to accept:

> *So the solution is also obvious: eat less, exercise more. The reason to question this conventional thinking is equally self-evident. The eat less / move more prescription has been widely disseminated for 40 years, and yet the prevalence of obesity, or the accumulation of unhealthy amounts of body fat, has climbed to unprecedented levels. Today more than a third of Americans are considered obese—more than twice the proportion of 40 years ago. Worldwide, more than half a billion people are now obese.*

In the end, we all want to know how to make the smartest choices at the supermarket. Merely counting calories based on food labels is an overly simplistic approach to eating a healthy diet—one that does not necessarily improve our health, even if it should help some of us to lose weight.

Instead we should think more carefully about the energy we get from our food in the context of human biology. Processed foods are so easily digested in the stomach and intestines that they give us a lot of energy for very little work. In contrast, veggies, nuts and whole grains make us sweat for our calories, generally offer far more vitamins and nutrients than processed items, and keep our gut bacteria happy. So it would be logical for people who want to eat healthier and forget the calories to favor whole and raw foods over highly processed foods.

GENETICALLY MODIFIED ORGANISMS (GMOS)

GMOs have a chapter dedicated to them because of their detrimental cause and effect on our overall health. Children's diseases are listed and show how they have grown over the years we have been fed genetically modified organisms.

NEURO IMMUNE DYSFUNCTION SYNDROME (NIDS)

Neuro Immune Dysfunction Syndrome (NIDS) refers to a group of illnesses that are the result of *acquired dysregulation* of both the immune system and the nervous system. They are *acquired disorders* that impact the body and the brain. Basically this means we create the disorders not inherit them.

Have you noticed that with each passing decade we have a new syndrome or disease that becomes prevalent in that space of time? Having begun practicing in the early 1970s, I have been dealing with all the various syndromes and/or diseases at one time or another. After a few years of the newest and hottest problem, I began to notice the similarity of symptoms.

How many new illnesses are there every 10 years? Is it possible they are the same diseases just given new names? In 2014, Health Science has come up with an explanation telling us that they are all a Neuroimmune disease. Neuroimmunology is the study of how the immune system and nervous system relate to one another in chronic conditions.

The brain and the digestive tract are considered our *first* and *second* brains. For example, when a person experiences mental stress, the brain responds by initiating 1400 different responses including the dumping of a variety of chemicals to our blood stream. This impacts the digestive system, and as a result, all of the body's systems.

Technically known as the enteric nervous system, the second brain consists of sheaths of neurons embedded in the walls of the long tube of our digestive system, which measures about nine meters end to end from the esophagus to the anus.

This multitude of neurons in the enteric nervous system enables us to "feel" the inner world of our gut and its contents. Much of this neural firepower comes to bear in the daily grind of digestion. Breaking down food, absorbing nutrients, and expelling of waste require chemical processing, mechanical mixing, and rhythmic muscle contractions that move everything on down the line.

Down the road, the blossoming field of Neurogastroenterology will likely offer some new insight into the workings of the second brain—and its impact on the body and mind.

CANCER

This topic has been a real concern to me as I have seen and read an increasing amount of misinformation on cancer in magazine articles, books, and the media. Now that we are in an age of instant information located on the Internet, there is often confusion between what is correct and incorrect. Do I believe I have all the answers? I will be very honest and say no. However, I am a cancer survivor for over 30 years and have spent many years studying the complexity of the human system to better understand how a human being physically operates.

That's why my heart goes out to so many who are desperate for good information. Many think because if it's in a book, it has to be true or if written by a health practitioner, it has to be accurate—when in truth, much is uneducated thoughts or theories. I use the word "theory" because it means it is an idea, but not scientifically proven or possible. As a believer in education, I am hoping to bring these myths to the forefront and through education help you learn to identify truth for the human's system.

SEVEN STAGES OF DISEASE

It has been my experience to witness fear, surprise, and utter confusion by a person receiving a negative diagnosis. Disease is never supposed to happen to us. We believe that this condition happened to us overnight and there was absolutely nothing that could have been done to spare us. Many of us feel like victims and completely without choice in this matter. I have been in this position more than once in my lifetime and understand the fear and feeling of helplessness. However, what I have since learned is there are choices, and most conditions do not happen overnight. The choices a person makes not to ever exercise, or to stop for lunch every day and eat fast foods, or lead a stressful, negative lifestyle can lead to the depletion and an imbalance of enzymes. Every one of us is born with an inherited ability to make metabolic enzymes. However, enzymes can either be repressed or destroyed when the body's condition or environment is not in balance.

It is these poor choices that we make. In fact, they result in the imbalances to the whole body, which allows disease to manifest. No, disease does not happen overnight. It takes years of this constant neglect and over-indulgence to alter our metabolic enzyme balance and create a disease condition. I wrote this many years ago for my thesis when I decided to quit studying disease and switched my degree from an M.D. to a Ph.D. in Health Sciences. My focus was on how a body works when in balance. By that I could then track ahead to the nature of a disease process. There are many cancer survivors like myself and there are things we have in common. One is education about our disease in order to stop our movement down that cancer slippery slope we were riding on. We did not want it to ride right into another organ and set up residence there. I hope you will recognize yourself in one of the stages and plan a way back to a healthier stage and into quality of life.

RENEWAL PROGRAM

This program is one I used in my clinics; it gives information so one begins healing at the cell itself. There is the beginning stage, which assists the body systems to begin recovery, and the second stage renews the cell itself. One needs to know when to feed or build the system and, just as important and possibly more so, when to fast. This program provides:

Knowledge of foods that will promote energy and renewal of our system

Knowledge of foods that will promote healthy tissue, bone, and muscle building

A plan for what to eat and how often

Exercise to refurbish the body and improve how we feel

Adequate pure water intake to bathe our cells and eliminate waste

Proper length of the program to allow for rebuilding—this will be anywhere from three to six weeks before moving into the Advanced Program.

Those that need the renewal program:

Anyone who is or has been out of balance (for an ongoing period of time), which has created imbalance within his or her body system itself such as:

Cancer patients

People diagnosed with conditions (system or organ dysfunction)

Obesity / overeating

Depression / anxiety

Fatigue / confusion

"Transformational Renewal" how to:

Renew and feel good while doing it

Know what takes place when you begin the renewal of all systems

Proper eating and exercise will promote energy throughout all systems of the body during each step of the Renewal Program

A simple one-page system for every day

PETS AND SUPPLEMENTAL DIGESTIVE ENZYMES

So many of us have pets and consider them a part of our family, and they have many of the same needs and disease as we humans. Most of the dog food we purchase contains ingredients our pets cannot effectively break down.

ATHLETIC PERFORMANCE AND RECOVERY

This chapter answers the question—Should athletes take supplemental digestive enzymes? You will read how some athletes answer this question.

LONGER HEALTHIER AND YOUTHFUL LIFE

You will find this a chapter for those who want to slow down the aging process. Obviously we will age, but how we do it many times is by our own choices. Quality of life is as important as slowing the aging process.

GUT BACTERIA AND FAT CELLS PRODUCE THE "PERFECT STORM" OF INFLAMMATION!

Chronic inflammation in your gut can disrupt the normal functioning of many bodily systems. There also appears to be a connection between certain types of bacteria and body fat, which produce a heightened inflammatory response and drives the inflammatory process. This wide array of health problems, including but not limited to obesity, insulin resistance, Type II diabetes, periodontal disease, stroke, and heart disease all have inflammation as a part of the disease.

Since the wide majority of Inflammatory diseases start in your gut, your diet and environmental factors affect your gut flora and disease. Diet accounts for about 80 percent of your health benefits and the running thread linking a wide variety of common health problems—from obesity and diabetes to heart disease and stroke—is chronic inflammation. Clearly, real key to reducing chronic inflammation in your body starts with your diet.

Microorganisms living in your digestive tract form a very important "inner ecosystem" that influences countless aspects of health. More specifically, the type and quantity of organisms in your gut interact with your body in ways that can either prevent or encourage the development of chronic inflammation, which is at the heart of many diseases, including heart disease and diabetes. The composition of your microflora may even dictate the ease with which you're able to shed unwanted pounds.

Contents

Appendix I

Appendix II

Chapter 1

The Miracle of Enzymes

JUST WHAT ARE ENZYMES, ANYWAY?

Although enzyme biochemistry has been the subject of intensive study since the 1930s, the role of enzymes in supplementation and therapy hasn't been widespread or understood by many people. Isn't it ironic that almost everyone knows the value of vitamins and minerals (co-enzymes) but cannot tell you anything about enzymes?

- Enzymes are necessary in every chemical reaction that occurs in our bodies
- All organs, tissues and 100 trillion cells in the body depend upon enzymes
- Co-enzymes (vitamins and minerals) require enzymes in order to be absorbed and used by the cell
- Enzyme utilization of co-enzymes create 100,000 chemical reactions every second for metabolism; allowing us to see, hear, feel, move, and think

Enzymes are proteins commonly referred to as metabolic enzymes when they are made in the body. They must be present before any chemical reaction can take place in our system. Even vitamins, minerals, and hormones cannot do their jobs without these enzymes. We used to say that enzymes were too small to be seen through the most powerful microscope. This has changed throughout the years with the stronger microscopes that allow us to see pictures of specific enzymes. Nevertheless, they are the catalysts (the spark or action), the dynamic power that gives us our ability to function at the highest level of good health.

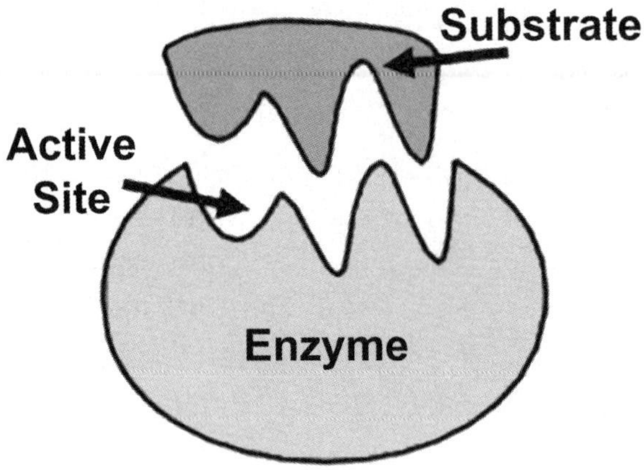

HOW DO OUR BODIES MAKE ENZYMES?

These delicate life-giving substances called enzymes are present in all living cells, whether vegetable or animal. Technically, enzymes are energized protein molecules. Our bodies can obtain them in only two ways—by making them inside the body (endogenous metabolic enzymes) or by acquiring them through the protein food we ingest from outside the body (exogenous enzymes) by using properly digested proteins to replenish or make more metabolic enzymes.

There are problems that occur with each source:

- As you get older, your body becomes much less efficient, thus producing significantly fewer enzymes than it did when young.
- Secondly, the greatest part of the food you eat today is genetically modified and your body does not recognize those unidentified proteins. The result of this is that you don't get enough proteins to replenish your supply of enzymes in order to remain healthy and energized.
- Furthermore, because enzymes are protein molecules, the body needs a constant supply of amino acids from our diets to continue replacing lost metabolic enzymes. If anyone at any age has a stomach digestive problem or does not consume enough protein in their diet, the body's ability to replenish its metabolic enzymes and rebuild is hindered.

Our bodies cannot exist without metabolic enzymes.

IF OUR BODIES MAKE THEIR OWN ENZYMES, WHY THEN DO WE NEED TO TAKE SUPPLEMENTAL DIGESTIVE ENZYMES?

A wide array of disorders can affect your digestive tract, a long tube of organs that begins at your mouth and ends at your anus. Over 90 million people suffer every day from some form of digestive issues (heartburn, acid reflux, GERD (gastro esophageal reflex disorder), IBS (irritable bowel syndrome), indigestion, constipation, diarrhea, abdominal pain, etc.).

- Your body produces digestive enzymes. However, it cannot produce enough digestive enzymes to keep up with the typical western diet, which is full of enzyme-depleted, cooked, and processed foods. This is one of the reasons why so many people suffer from digestive-related health problems.
- Add to this fact that genetically modified foods cannot be broken down properly and seen by the immune system as an allergy. Eighty percent of our immune system is located in our digestive tract.
- If you were not breastfed as an infant and/or given solid food too early in life would make you a likely candidate.
- As we age our ability to produce digestive enzymes decreases by 13 percent every 10-year period.
- If you suffer from gluten sensitivities.
- If you have been diagnosed with a disease.

There are some diseases that are marked by an abnormal response by the body's immune system. Normally, the immune cells protect the body from infection. In some people however, the immune system mistakes food, bacteria, and other materials in the intestine for foreign substances, and it attacks the cells of the intestines. In the process, the body sends white blood cells into the lining of the intestines where they produce chronic inflammation.

We need enzymes when we eat food that has been produced with genetically modified organisms. Such foods are referred to as "Frankenfood" or the foods that our bodies no longer recognize. GMO refers to a process that scientists use to make food sources using animals, insects, virus, bacteria, and human DNA. I will cover this in another chapter along with synthetic foods like sugars and fat. Pink synthetic meat . . . ugh!

In his book *Enzyme Nutrition*, written 30 years ago, Dr. Edward Howell tells of research done at the University of Toronto. The research showed that each child is born with a definite amount of enzyme potential that can be saved or wasted. It can be used up fast or sparingly, according to one's life tempo. Also, this enzyme potential can last longer when reinforced with enzyme supplements.

OUR OWN DNA TELLS US WHEN TO MAKE DIGESTIVE ENZYMES

While yet an embryo (less than 5 days old), we receive an estimated 20,000 to 25,000 genes carrying 3 billion bits of genetic information. This information constitutes an instruction book for his or her body's proteins. This information is stored in our genes and the DNA carries it. What this tells us is that we are first given instruction on how to handle our proteins. Enzymes themselves are proteins.

While yet a fetus in Mother's womb between the 9th and 12th week, we are given our ability to develop digestive enzymes (enzyme potential) that lasts for a lifetime. These three weeks are very important and if the mother is healthy and digesting properly, we have a more improved possibility. Some mothers don't even know they are pregnant and are in just the first trimester of their pregnancy. I am not going to go through all the possibilities that can go wrong but please know that my second child came in to this world with enzyme deficiencies. It took me years to understand this. From this time, I began developing enzyme therapy and teaching supplemental digestive enzymes to practitioners.

What does my time as a fetus or baby have to do with my digestion now?

- We first make digestive enzymes (enzyme potential) while in our mother's womb during our 9th to 12th week.
- This enzyme potential is to last throughout our life.
- The only digestive enzyme turned on at birth is meant for our own Mother's breast milk.
- This remains so for at least **18 months** and then babies may begin to slowly digest some carbohydrates added in their diet.
- It is not until they are around **36 months old** and have begun to cut 12 to 14 teeth will they be able to utilize natural sugars in foods.
- They will need the teeth for chewing as well as grinding, and the environment of their gut will then be able to handle natural sugars.
- This is all dependent on the genes instruction and directing their DNA as to when to turn on their digestive enzymes.

TIME OUT FOR A MINUTE! WHY HAVEN'T I HEARD THIS ABOUT ENZYMES?

If you are like many who have first heard me speak enthusiastically about the endless roles played by enzymes, you are beginning to wonder why you have not seen or heard much press coverage about them. You will also wonder why we were not instructed during pregnancy on the importance of enzymes and foods for our babies. Of late, the biggest coverage is on raw foods supplying enzymes, and I believed this was true for years. I wrote about it in my previous book. However, as I did further research, I found that labs measuring them in fecal matter and urine could measure the food-produced enzymes. Universities such as Wright State University wrote that the food enzymes were present but they had not been utilized. They went further to use patients with colon bags to see if there was different information, but the food-produced enzymes were still dormant.

But how many true enzyme specialists do you know? Most of these specialists have a degree in enzymology. Furthermore, would the prospect of reading a newspaper article or watching a TV documentary on scientific enzymes fill you with excitement? Probably not, yet the healing power of enzymes has been documented for decades. When correctly used, these enzymes can do wonders for our minds and bodies. We have briefly touched on the importance of enzymes for good digestion, and Chapter Two will cover Biochemical Individualism (scientific word for body typing) and specific needs for enzymes in more detail.

You are probably reading this book for one of two reasons. You care enough about your own health or someone who cares about you gave it to you. No matter which way you came to read about enzymes, you would definitely understand how they work and why they are so important when you read this book. There are many enzyme products on the market today, each with its own purpose.

ENERGIZE YOUR LIFE WITH NATURE'S LIFESAVERS

These wonderful little lifesavers serve your body in two important and distinctly different ways. First, they break down the nutrients contained in the food into chemical substances that are fine enough to pass through the lining of the digestive tract cells. From there, they enter the blood stream. The entire process is fascinating, and I plan to cover it in more detail in another chapter. Your body considers digestion as its most important duty. When a newly eaten meal enters the stomach, digestive enzymes are released from all systems of the body to initiate digestion process. However, this same enzyme energy is also needed elsewhere to repair, regulate, and reactivate the other systems of the body. These systems have no choice but to partially shut down during digestion. The other alternative is to supplement your diet with digestive enzyme supplements. This will be covered extensively in another chapter.

The other major role of enzymes is to keep the metabolism working at full throttle. This includes burning fats, making and feeding cells, and releasing energy wherever needed. Every bodily function, from building new skin, muscle, bone, glands, and nerves to those that rid the system of toxins, depend completely on enzymatic activity. Skin glowing with health, an efficiently operating colon, liver, heart, and brain, fully functioning lungs, kidneys and hormones all rely on enzymes. It can truly be said that enzymes are Nature's lifesavers!

WHAT ARE SOME COMMON SOURCES OF ENZYMES?

Metabolic enzymes are those produced by the body. They are necessary for life itself. Age and high stress reduce our ability to produce necessary enzymes. Eighty percent of your body's own digestive process expends energy. If you are run down, under stress, living in a very hot or very cold climate, pregnant, or a frequent air traveler, are you aware that your body may require enormous quantities of enzymes? Because our entire system functions through enzymatic action, we must supplement our enzymes. Aging deprives us of our ability to produce necessary enzymes. The medical profession tells us that all diseases are caused by a lack or imbalance of enzymes. Our very lives are dependent upon them!

Food enzymes are preserved intact in raw foods. Uncooked fruit and vegetables contain their own enzymes. A ripening banana is a good example of how raw-food enzymes work. The banana transforms itself from a hard, starchy plant into a very soft, brown and sweet one through a process requiring energy from its enzymes. Their plant enzymes work first to take in nutrients and then allow them to ripen with the same enzyme process. There is confusion in the raw food world over the enzymes that raw foods contain. These food enzymes are specifically for the food itself to obtain their own nutrients from the soil, tree, or host they grow on.

If you eat raw fruits or vegetables, their specific enzymes can be used to mix with our metabolic or supplemental enzymes to better gain the nutrients in food. Food enzymes when in a raw state can sometimes make it to the small intestine before becoming dormant. They do not stand in place of our own metabolic enzymes, but they work in food by opening the door to the nutrients. However, if the food is heated by cooking, the heating process kills the food enzymes and many of their nutrients. They then are not available during human digestion because they are destroyed in heating and/or further made dormant in the environment of the human stomach. We may juice these raw foods, but the friction of the juicer limits their enzymes. Food enzymes were created to work for their own needs. Such enzymes are not available for our enzymatic needs as in providing human enzymes. The process of raw foods enzymes during digestion is referred to as synergism. Some raw foods such as nuts, beans, and grains contain enzyme inhibitors. These foods need to be roasted or prepared to kill off the inhibitors, which can cause an inhibiting of digestion in the human stomach.

Supplemental plant-based digestive enzymes are the third source for these miraculous substances. They are grown on plant foods (as their host) in a laboratory where they are fed to become whatever digestive enzyme is required, but they do not contain their host. The host is a plant source and its use is just a platform to host the mycelial or biochemical enzymes. When mature, the fungus is removed and the remainder is a pure fluid that is dried to a fine powder substance. They are known as plant enzymes but they are really mycelial or microbial produced bio-identical enzymes to the human body. Enzymes cannot be made like synthetic vitamins and minerals. They must be grown in plant form and extracted without chemicals in a laboratory process. Supplemental plant-based enzymes are usually sold in capsule form. They are swallowed with food to assist in the digestion of a particular meal. They work throughout the entire digestive system, from esophagus to rectum.

Animal enzymes, sometimes known as glandular enzymes, are the other enzymes available for human consumption. For instance, **pancreatin** comes from the pancreas of a slaughterhouse hog or ox. Pancreatin requires an alkaline pH setting to work. It begins working in the latter stages of the digestive process in the small intestine. The reason for this is that they are proteins and therefore would be broken down in the stomach. Because of this, they require an enteric coating for time release and are usually found in tablet or capsule form. Their best work is in the alkaline setting of the blood but not necessarily for digestive purposes. Animal produced enzymes are not recommended for children or pregnant women due to their coating.

Plant enzymes are **bromelain**, a proteolytic enzyme and a milk-clotting enzyme derived from the pineapple stem, and **papain**, an enzyme derived from the papaya tree. They were first used as meat tenderizers and ingredients in beer until they became more refined to be used in supplements. **Pepsin** is an enzyme involved in the breakdown of proteins in the stomach and in the recent past was usually prepared from the stomach of pigs and required an acid pH setting. Kiwi has some value in breaking down fiber and some dairy products. There are some who experience bowel irritation from the use of papain and kiwi that is similar to the bloating from eating at salad bars.

Plant-based supplemental digestive enzymes have the ability to aid digestion throughout the entire digestive process. Therefore, these enzymes are more useful to the body's digestion than any other type of enzyme supplement. Now let's look at *industrial grade enzymes*, such as those used in cleaning agents. These enzymes act as grease-eaters. In this category, there are other single purpose enzymes designed to do one specific thing, such as breaking down a particular type of grease. There are also *commercial grade enzymes*. These are sold in large quantities and are used for baking, tanning leather, or fermenting the malt used to brew beer.

The focus of this book is *nutritional pharmaceutical grade plant-based enzymes*. These have a broader spectrum of use and come in a more purified and stable form. I have studied these types of enzymes more extensively. Personally, I use only these enzymes. Here are my reasons for doing so. I wish I could say that all packaged, nutritional enzymes are completely free of contaminants. Sad to say, that is not the case. Some companies do not use the purest products so that they can sell at lower prices. The enzymes I use are those grown for a specific function—efficient digestion by a human. I am not interested in those commercial grade enzymes found in the bakeries and breweries. I recommend that anyone genuinely concerned with improving his or her health should avoid them as well. Many of you have not had access to a high-quality source. I have met users of enzymes who have had adverse reactions to them. This is generally because these product fillers are impure. Some kind of filler has been used to allow the manufacturers to sell at lower prices. Only those enzymes with no fillers should be ingested to ensure your maximum health and well-being. If it is necessary for you to take those with fillers, make sure the fillers come from a product that contains nutrients. It is a well-known fact that not everything is "natural" even if labeled that way.

Synthetic vitamins can be legally labeled "natural" if they contain a small amount of natural food ingredients. People often think they are taking high dosages of absolutely pure vitamins or enzymes from an "all-natural" source. The truth is that if these high-strength capsules were derived entirely from a perfectly pure, natural food source, one of them would be the size of a table not a tablet. That would be difficult to swallow! This is why I want the public to be aware of what they are getting from their investment. This comes up when those formulating the tablets are mixing enzymes that work in a higher pH than the human body.

Plant based enzyme supplements can be purchased from health food stores, through multi-level marketing groups or mail order, and from health care professionals. They will vary in strength, ingredients, and the amount of fillers they contain. There are even claims that certain vitamins or foods are enzymes. Do not confuse plant-based enzymes with those made from animal products. Of all enzymes used for increasing our level of good health, it is important to be aware of a substandard enzyme supplement that may not work sufficiently in the human body. Remember, each of them works differently and may be intended for something other than digestion.

CAREFUL... WATCH IT! OH, NEVER MIND... 10 MILLION OF YOUR CELLS JUST DIED!

To illustrate the importance of enzymes, did you know that in less time than it takes you to read this sentence, and well before you finish the paragraph, 10 million of your cells have died? Are you aware that there are at least 100 trillion cells at work in your body right now? Scientists have identified that there are at least 9,000 different protease enzymes alone in the human body. It takes 13,000 enzymes to make just one cell! There are 20,000 enzymes in each human cell that perform 100,000 different chemical actions every second!

Enzymes are pure proteins. They are catalysts in the combination of different molecules. Without them, a single cell consisting of more than one hundred thousand different chemicals could not exist. Your DNA molecules receive their ability to do all the tasks on the cellular level because of the presence of enzymes. As I stated earlier, the required nutrients our bodies use to make metabolic enzymes come from the food we eat. That is, if we digest our food thoroughly and use the nutrients efficiently.

Forty-five nutrients (in their proper amounts) derived from the food we eat nourish each and every cell.

These nutrients are:

- 19 minerals, in prescribed amounts
- 13 vitamins
- 9 amino acids
- 1 protein (nitrogen)
- 1 fat
- 1 water
- 1 glucose
- Plus 20,000 enzymes

WAY TO GO... YOU JUST MADE BILLIONS! (OF RED BLOOD CELLS THAT IS...)

When I suggest that there is an exact amount of vitamins and minerals needed to maximize good health, I mean that mega-dosing can create more problems than consuming few nutrients in some instances. What regulates all this is the delivery of enzymes. For example, there are billions of red blood cells made from bone marrow each second. In order to build these red blood cells, a form of iron called heme iron is necessary. We need to eat protein foods in order to obtain heme iron. However, if the protein food is not properly digested, our bodies will not extract the nutrients required. Inefficiencies in our digestive system typically allow only about 15 percent of the heme iron present in animal proteins, and only about 3 percent of the heme iron present in plant foods, to be absorbed by our bodies. Improving the efficiency of the digestive system is vital to obtaining nutrients such as hemi-iron. Digestive enzymes are what allow the body to properly digest and assimilate the nutrients we consume. If your intake of calcium is too low, you will experience hair loss and brittle finger and toe nails. You will also show all the symptoms of those who have bone problems. Too much calcium can form bone spurs and cause blood disorders. What happens when you do not have enough enzymatic action in your body? Once again, it takes most of our energy just to digest our food. Digestive enzymes are the delivery mechanism in the body. Not only do they assist in the breakdown of our food, but also deliver the nutrients to every part of the body.

Absorption cells called *villi* are present in the small intestine to aid in digestion. If all the villi in your body were laid out end to end, they would measure about half the length of a football field. Villi replace their cells every two days. With aging, we lose our ability to replace these cells, so they can no longer absorb nutrients for delivery to other cells. Where an imbalance occurs, such as Celiac disease, the villi fold over and are not able to absorb the nutrients. The next step is that undigested food, such as protein, begins to clog the system. Remember, undigested protein begins to putrefy and will eventually cause health problems. The importance of proper digestion is mind-boggling. Every function must be perfectly synchronized with every other function. When we lack a particular enzyme, vitamin, or mineral, the resulting imbalance causes diseases. We are now considering the following facts due to the unhealthy eating habits that dominate our society: If you have digestive problems, you will have trouble rebuilding cells, which leads to an array of health disorders. My own experience in working with medical doctors and researchers has proved this to be true. You may think it is too simplistic to conclude that illness is caused by inadequate digestion, but I am convinced this is true.

LOOK AT YOURSELF IN THE MIRROR—YOU ARE LOOKING AT YOUR CELL PARTS!

You are made up of cells. If you look at yourself in a mirror you are actually looking at your cell parts. An adult body (dependent on your size and age) is made up of 100 trillion cells. For example, when you look at your little finger, you will recognize that it holds one to two billion cells within it alone. Cells are not large. They may be shaped slightly different from each other (organ cells to red blood cells) but the thing in common is that they are all cells and require the same enzymes and oxygen to work.

ENZYMES

At any given moment, enzymes are doing all of the work being done inside any cell. If you understand enzymes, you understand cells. **A human cell has about 20,000 different types of enzymes** floating around in the cytoplasm (gel-like substance holding the cell together) like a bag.

Enzymes have extremely interesting properties that make them little chemical-reaction machines. The purpose of an enzyme in a cell is to allow the cell to carry out chemical reactions very quickly. As an example, the enzymes utilize nutrients and produce **100,000 different chemical actions every second**. These reactions allow the cell to build things or take things apart as needed. This is how a cell grows and reproduces. At the most basic level, a cell is really a little bag full of chemical reactions that are made possible by enzymes!

Enzymes in your body are made from **amino acids and they are proteins**. Amino acids string together in bunches of 100 to 1,000 in a very specific and unique order so as to form an enzyme. The chain of amino acids then folds into a unique shape. That shape allows the enzyme to carry out specific chemical reactions—an enzyme acts as a very efficient catalyst for a specific chemical reaction. The enzyme tremendously speeds up that reaction.

You may have heard of people who are **lactose intolerant**, or you may suffer from this problem yourself. The problem arises because the sugar in milk (lactose) does not get broken down into its glucose components. Therefore, it cannot be digested. The intestinal cells do not have the lactase available for lactose-intolerant people. Lactase is the enzyme required to break down lactose. This problem shows how the lack of just one enzyme in the human body can lead to problems. However, a lactose intolerant person can swallow a capsule with lactase prior to drinking milk and the problem is solved.

Inside a cell, there are around 20,000 types of enzymes (lactase being just one of them). All of the enzymes float freely in the cytoplasm (gel-like substance in the cell membrane), waiting for the chemical (nutrient) they recognize to float by so they can utilize it. There are hundreds or millions of copies of each different type of enzyme, depending on how important a reaction is to a cell and how often the reaction is required. These enzymes do everything from breaking glucose down for energy, to building cell walls, constructing new enzymes, and allowing the cell to reproduce. Enzymes do all of the work inside cells, and it takes 13,000 enzymes just to build one human cell.

MAKING ENZYMES THE MIRACLE OF LIFE

As long as a cell's membrane is intact and it is making all of the enzymes it needs to function properly, the cell is **"alive."** The enzymes it needs to function properly allow the cell to create energy from glucose, construct the pieces that make up its cell wall, reproduce and of course, produce new enzymes. I do want to mention that if it does not have what it needs, the cell will die (implode). This is called hemolysis.

RECOMMENDATIONS:

And how does the cell produce them when it needs them? If a cell is just a collection of enzymes causing chemical reactions that make the cell do what it does, then how can a set of chemical reactions create the necessary enzymes, and how can the cell reproduce? Where does the miracle of life come from?

At the beginning of our lives while yet just an embryo (within the very beginning of our life), we are given an instruction book specific for each one of us. This instruction book contains an estimated 20,000 to 25,000 genes carrying 3 billion bits of genetic information instructing our DNA just how it is to make our proteins (enzymes) for life.

The answer to these questions lies in the DNA, which guides the cell in its production of new enzymes. DNA is a carrier of genetic information. Think about it as just a working model made up of four different parts. Now imagine a set of blocks that has only four different shapes, or an alphabet that has only four different letters. DNA is a long string of blocks or letters that spells out your given information.

A human's DNA is about 3 billion blocks long. Just so you can get an idea of what that means, it is the equivalent to nearly 70 trips from the earth to the sun and back. It is tightly wrapped into 23 structures called chromosomes. This ensures that the DNA is packed tightly in order to fit inside a cell. The amazing thing to me is that the DNA is nothing more than a self-replicating pattern or recipe that tells the cell how to make its proteins! That is all that DNA does. It carries the template (instructions) on how to form an enzyme. If you were to unravel your DNA, it would stretch from here to the moon!

ENZYMES AT WORK

There are all sorts of enzymes at work inside the human cells, and many of them are incredibly interesting! Cells use enzymes internally to grow, reproduce, create energy, rid the cell of waste, and they often excrete enzymes outside their cell walls as well.

Energy enzymes - A set of 10 different enzymes allow a cell to perform glycolysis. Another eight enzymes control the Krebs cycle (citric-acid cycle). These two processes together allow a cell to turn **glucose and oxygen into ATP** (adenosine triphosphate) **energy!** In an oxygen-consuming human cell, one glucose molecule forms 36 ATP molecules. ATP is the fuel that is able to power enzymes by performing chemical reactions.

DNA-manipulation enzymes - They are specialized enzymes that move along DNA strands and repair them. There are other enzymes that can untwist DNA strands to reproduce them (DNA polymerase). DNA polymerase is our most accurate or valuable enzyme, for a good reason. It is the keeper of our most precious resource: our genetic information. DNA polymerase takes our DNA, gently unwinds it, and builds a complementary mate to each strand. Still other enzymes can find small patterns on DNA and attach to them, blocking access to that section of DNA (DNA-binding proteins).

Enzyme-production enzymes - All of these enzymes have to come from somewhere, so there are enzymes that produce the cell's enzymes! RNA (Ribonucleic acid), in three different forms (named messenger RNA, transfer RNA, and ribosomal RNA), is a big part of the process.

Supplemental oral enzymes – We ingest these enzymes with a meal known as supplemental digestive enzymes to assist in the proper digestion of foods. For proper digestion to take place, four major and three minor digestive enzymes are required. The carbohydrate-splitting enzymes are called by many different names depending on the food they break down. For example, the first enzyme that was ever recognized by Biochemistry Science many years ago was **amylase**. This enzyme aids in the digestion of starches such as potatoes, pasta, and bread. **Cellulase** breaks down cellulose (the fiber found in vegetables and other plant materials). However, the body does not produce cellulase. Hence, the synthetic commercial fiber we ingest for the purpose of scouring the colon of unassimilated matter often fosters more intestinal problems. Undigested fiber leaves wax like residue in the small intestine. This ends up causing absorption maladies in the small intestine. This is why we ingest cellulase even though the body does not produce it. The most widely known of all the enzymes is **lactase**. It breaks down the milk sugar lactose. If the body is not producing lactase (lactase deficiency), the lactose in milk is not broken down, resulting in digestive problems. Additionally, some dairy products can cause allergies because of casein (the protein) in milk. Other lesser-known enzymes that break down carbohydrates are **invertase**, **sucrose**, and **maltase**, which break down simple sugars. There are nine other different carbohydrate-splitting enzymes that break down the rest of the carbohydrate foods such as fruits and other vegetables. Poorly digested carbohydrates/starches can ferment in the large intestine, creating gas and other symptoms of discomfort. **Protease** enzymes digest proteins such as red meats, fowl, fish, and nuts. If improperly digested protein putrefies in the large intestine, it will cause indigestion toxicity and smelly gas. **Lipase** enzymes break down lipids (fats / triglycerides) and are required for balancing fatty acids. Fats that are not thoroughly digested turn rancid in the system and create pungent odors and poor cholesterol balance. Is it any wonder that we are an entire society suffering from constipation, gas, indigestion, and halitosis?

Besides the rancid gases that can be caused by poor digestion, our vitamins cannot be properly absorbed in the cells without enzymes. Carbohydrate-splitting enzymes assist in absorption of water-soluble nutrients such as B vitamins and vitamin C. Protein-splitting enzymes assist in amino acids, our building blocks of the body. On the other hand, fat-splitting enzymes are responsible for the delivery of fat-soluble vitamins such as vitamin D, E, or K.

A cell really is nothing but a set of chemical reactions, and enzymes make those reactions happen properly!

IS THERE A WAY TO KNOW WHAT ENZYMES ARE DEFICIENT IN MY BODY?

The obvious symptoms of poor digestion are burps and belches, excessive gas, heartburn, nausea, constipation, feeling tired after eating, or an allergic reaction to a particular food. Another way to discover a deficiency is through observing which foods you crave or eat the most. These include caffeine, chocolate, refined sugars, and cooked or processed foods. The only tests for enzymes lost are when an organ is stressed and is losing its enzymes such as our pancreas, heart, or liver. I am not aware of any other test for enzymes deficiencies, but questionnaires can be used to find more information on this. I mentioned earlier that there are labs that can observe the enzymes lost in the fecal matter or urine. But these have been food enzymes. When an enzyme is working, it is used up and then converted into amino acids. Think about this with me – if it takes 13,000 enzymes to create just one cell, and every cell in your body (all 100 trillion) requires 20,000 enzymes each, then it would be impossible to measure "lack" of enzymes.

I refer you to Chapter Two for further information on enzyme deficiencies. This might be the right time to determine your biochemical type (similar to body type). There are four basic types, each associated with a specific enzyme deficiency.

TESTIMONIALS

***"Your company** has very well saved my life. I had to go through ten brands of enzymes before your digestive product helped me. In a few days, I am sleeping better, my diabetes is normalizing and even the natural curl on my hair I had lost is returning. You are right on target, realizing that many persons needing digestive enzymes could also be suffering from a very sensitive stomach and with gastric conditions, thus need gentle, pure and special enzyme formula. I will tell everyone that needs enzymes about yours. I will be forever grateful to your company!" - Tina M.*

***"No, I haven't dropped off the planet!** But, all of a sudden I got real busy—which may reveal a lot, as I am feeling better than I have in years. I added a couple of diet changes you recommended, digestive enzymes and Probiotics. In other words, small changes made a big difference!" - Jeff S. - Garland, TX*

***"Actually Dr. DicQie Fuller-Looney** is the writer and she formulated a lot of our products!!!! I know her personally. She is awesome! And I've learned so much from her. Love it :) that's awesome! Glad you read her book!" - Angely R. - Bronx, NY*

***"Wow!! I admire you and your work,** it's really great to finally know the woman behind this great project!! I Really thank you because you changed my life!" - Jessica R - Villahermosa, Tabasco*

Chapter 2

What is Your Body (Biochemical) Type?

WHAT WORKS FOR ONE DOES NOT WORK FOR ALL

Have you noticed how people appear to be one of four basic shapes? At any shopping mall in the Midwest, for example, it is not unusual to observe many shoppers who carry most of their weight in their tummy or upper torso, but not their buttocks. A cowboy who has trouble holding up his jeans because his hips are smaller than his tummy falls into this category. You will also see women with large breasts and shoulders but have small flat buttocks. On the West Coast, health-conscious men and women tend to carry their weight evenly all over their bodies. They would rather have fatigue problems than suffer from weight problems. In the East, many people, especially women, have large hips wider than the shoulders and oversized thighs.

You will also find people whose body shapes mature later than others everywhere. These types have boyish or childlike shapes. This does not mean that these shapes are peculiar to specific geographic locations. However, when a particular nationality is concentrated in one state, this often accounts for a preponderance of one of the body types in that locality. We inherit our body shapes, with their strengths and weaknesses, from our ancestors.

What does this have to do with you, or this book? Everything, because different body shapes come with different needs and different enzyme needs. The key word is "different." This difference makes it impossible to have one perfect food or diet that works for everyone.

Now as you think about these varied body shapes, consider the distinct cravings that go along with each of them. One person may be drawn to very sweet foods, while another strongly dislikes desserts. Another may prefer a good steak rather than a slice of chocolate fudge cake. Doctors ask their patients about their own health and that of their families. These doctors are very aware that certain weaknesses and disorders are inherited and various medications and foods affect people very differently.

Dating back to the ancient Egyptians, over thirty-four books have been written on the subject of body typing. For example, Ayurvedic medicine, originating in India 5,000 years ago, is completely based on doshas or the way we are driven to different tastes whether salty, sour, or sweet. Problem has been that not everyone fits the three medical types known as ectomorph, endomorph, or mesomorph. Nor do you fit in the ancient Ayurvedic types known by their dosha tastes as Vata, Pitta, or Kapha. Because of this they have altered their three types, which now includes a mixed type. Last is our American Apple, Pear, or Banana and/or triangle, inverted triangle, or rectangle. This does not mean you do not fit anywhere since there are countries you are very prevalent.

As you may see, the study or biochemical science of body typing is not new. Health professionals have always been very aware of the differences, and similarities, in body types and muscle tones. I believe that one of the major reasons why any body type suffers weaknesses and gets out of balance is due to enzyme deficiencies. These are inherited and compounded through poor eating habits and stress on the system.

TESTIMONIALS

> *"I thought I would let you know that a patient called me and said she has already lost 7 lbs. on her new program. She has had such a struggle with losing weight and she is really excited about these results. She said she got into her 'skinny pants' this week. She said they were still a little tight, but she wore them anyway. She said she has not been able to get into them for 3.5 years! She is really staying on the body type diet and the enzymes. She is still excited about the results and I know she will continue. Thank you again for your help!" - Mamie W., ND*

> *"After attending your Biochemical Individualism seminar for doctors I took your recommendations to heart, so much so that when I arrived home I met with my entire staff. Understand first that things were not running as they should in a large practice like mine. The problems extended from proper daily flow to finances. Recognizing each one of my staff's biochemical types helped me understand their strength and weaknesses. I moved the nurse (Type Two) who was at the front desk to assist me and answer our patient's questions. I moved the other nurse (Type One), who had been assisting me, to the front desk to welcome*

the patients and take payment. The financial person (Type Three) moved to manager overseeing the running of the office. I then hired a financial person (Type Four) to make sure all the details of insurance and billing statements were accurate. Our morning meetings' food was changed to fit their types, and we are exploding with energy and balance. Dr. Fuller, I know you are thinking, 'Only a Type Three would do this!'" - William M., MD - Atlanta, GA

HOW YOUR OWN BODY SHAPE AFFECTS YOU AND YOUR LOVED ONES

All four of the basic body types have certain weaknesses common to all of them. You, but not necessarily the other members of your family may carry the greater part of your weight in your upper torso and tummy. Your buttocks may be flat and your legs are strong. Quite probably, you are a family member that enjoys meat as the main part of your meals. You and those like you in your family could very well suffer from lower back problems, acidic stomach, pain in the left shoulder, constipation, stress, reflex, and high blood pressure.

For those in a family whose weight tends to be evenly distributed all over, you will find hypoglycemia, low blood pressure, eczema, allergies, colon problems, anxiety, and fatigue to be common ailments among them. You gravitate toward sweets, breads, pasta, and chocolate. If you gain weight, it will invariably be carried in your face and throughout your body including the size of your feet. Lastly it will be in your buttocks and abdominal area. You work harder than others to maintain muscle mass. However, remember not everyone in the family may be exactly alike.

Those members who enjoy tasty, strong flavored foods like ethnic foods, wine, ice cream, heavily-spiced food, or lots of salt and pepper have their own set of disorders. One or all of you may suffer from kidney problems, hormone imbalance, enlarged prostate, skin irritations, sinus and mucous trouble, cysts, gallbladder distress, or indigestion that might include constipation to diarrhea. Your muscle mass is mostly below the waist.

The other, and one of the most interesting body types, is the type for one in which the family has serious difficulties with lactose intolerance. The cause of this is enzyme deficiencies of lactase, yet they have serious cravings for all dairy products. Some of the common maladies of this type are milk allergies, other allergies that range from foods to airborne microorganisms, spastic colon, aching joints—especially the knees—and a continuous feeling of exhaustion for no reason. If you have this body type, you carry the least amount of muscle mass on your body. The benefit of this particular type is that you are one of the youngest looking members of your family.

QUIZ: WHAT BODY TYPE ARE YOU?

In these descriptions, do you recognize yourself or someone you know? Are any of these families yours? Do you feel you belong in each one of these categories? If you answered, "yes" to any of these questions, and you will, it is because we inherit our body types from our parents. If your parents married outside of their own nationality, you will probably have a combined or overlapping body type. For instance, an Irish man and an Italian woman get married and have a family. We know that the Irish are evenly shaped and love sugar, potatoes, and alcohol. Italians, on the other hand, are known for their curves and indulging in rich, strong-flavored, and highly seasoned starchy foods. The child will always have some of the strengths and weaknesses of both parents. The Italian mother will cook foods she likes and see to it that her husband has an ample supply of breads and desserts. This may all sound delicious to you— it certainly does to me! However, as an adult, a child from this marriage has developed a weak immune system due to the stressful job he has. And he will seek the help of a nutritionist.

What are his best food choices? Should he be a vegetarian? These are the exact questions I had to answer when I became a health care professional. I realized very early that what works for one does not necessarily work for another. There is a very good reason for this. We are not all the same biochemical body type nor do we have the same needs and strengths.

FOUR MAIN BODY (BIOCHEMICAL) TYPES

I will refer to the four body types by numbers. It is not that one is more important than another. I have worked with body typing for over 30 years and I find it is best to begin with the category in which I saw the greatest number of body types where I lived. This is not Texas where I currently live, otherwise the types and the numbers would be different.

Questionnaire: If six or more of the 12 characteristics listed apply to you, then that is your category or ruling body type. Your food choices may not be the best for your health and may be the source of many of your health problems. However, you continue to crave them, but you do not break them down properly. In conventional medical practice, the body types are referred to by the name of the gland that rules each one.

BODY (BIOCHEMICAL) TYPE ONE

Type One is known as Para for the parathyroid or thyroid gland. This type is defined by the following traits:

- The widths of your clavicles and your hipbones are the same.
- Your waist may have a bit of a midriff bulge because of the tipping of your hipbones.
- You have high perky buttocks.
- You gain weight evenly, from the top of your head to your toes.
- If overweight, your excess fat is in the stomach and waist area. Men have "spare tire," women hold fat in their buttocks.
- You crave sugar in the form of desserts, breads, pastas, fruits, and vegetables.
- You are drawn to chocolate for fat and sugar mix.
- You get fatigued by midday and sometimes get up tired.
- You suffer depression or mood swings.
- You often have cold hands or feet.
- If you are female, you get PMS.
- Your blood pressure is on the low side.
- You have experienced hypoglycemia.
- Allergies are common for you.
- You are prone to eczema or skin rash

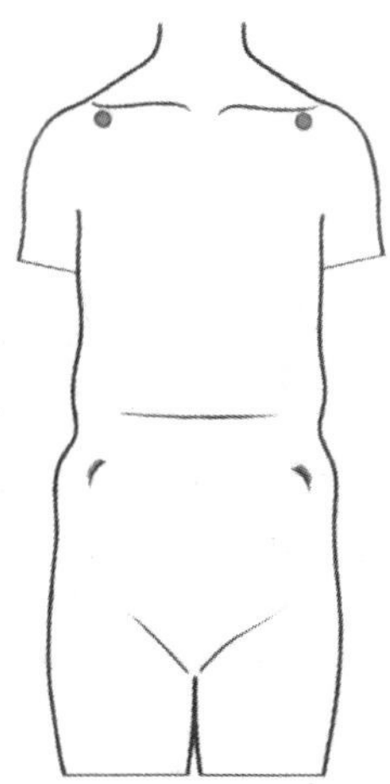

BODY (BIOCHEMICAL) TYPE TWO

Type Two is known as the Estro or Testro biochemical body type. The controlling glands for type twos are the gonadal system. The following list of traits defines this body type. Again, if six or more of these apply to you, this is your body type category:

- The width of your clavicle is shorter than the width of your hipbone. Your buttocks are low slung.
- In women, the greater part of the weight is in the buttocks and upper thighs. You wear a small top to a larger bottom in clothes.
- In men, your excess weight is in the abdominal region and lower body.
- Male or female your legs are generally strong in comparison to the upper part of your body.
- Your favorite foods are tasty, or strong-flavored such as spiced, creamed, salty, peppered, or smoked foods.
- You prefer to drink wine or a beverage other than water with your meals.
- Your favorite desserts are rich, like ice cream or chocolate.
- You enjoy fried fish, chicken, onion rings, and French fries.
- You like Italian, Oriental, and Mexican cuisines.
- You suffer from indigestion (bloating or gas) where your ribs come together.
- Gallbladder problems are common.
- You are bothered by kidney and bladder infections.
- You have a tendency toward cysts, dermatitis, or skin disorders.

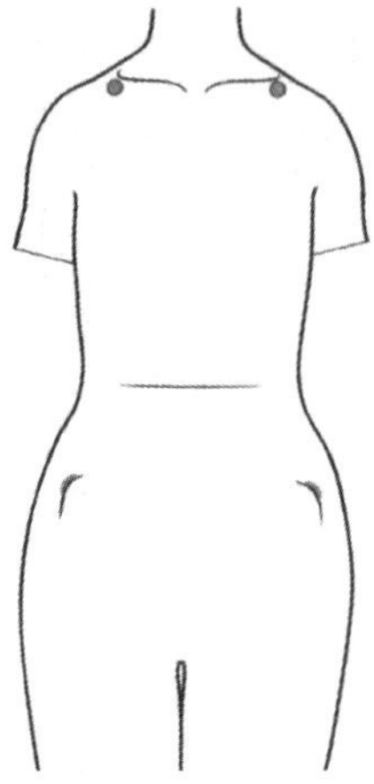

BODY (BIOCHEMICAL) TYPE THREE

The third type is known as Supra, for the suprarenal or adrenal glands. This type is defined by the following traits:

- Your clavicles are much wider than the width of your hip bones.
- You are able to build muscle quite easily.
- You carry your weight in your tummy and upper torso including your back.
- Your buttocks are fairly flat and do not have shape unless you are working out.
- Your legs are strong and firm at any age.
- A meal is not complete for you without meat or some kind of protein.
- You salt or season your food without tasting it first.
- You gravitate to all proteins: lunch meats, sausage, fish, poultry, nuts, cheese, and eggs.
- You suffer from stiff joints or pain in your left shoulder.
- You must drink at least one beverage with your meal.
- You have hypertension or high blood pressure.
- You feel stressed rather than fatigued.
- Constipation is a big problem for you.
- Gas, flatulence, or bloating is a way of life for you.
- You prefer stimulation from what you eat, drink, or think.

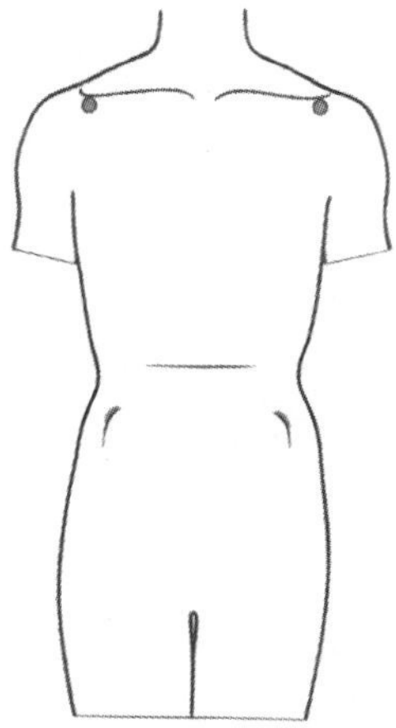

BODY (BIOCHEMICAL) TYPE FOUR

The fourth type is known as Neuro. It gets its name from the neurological and endocrine systems. These glands control the hormone production of other glands and indirectly affect the neurological (nervous system). The width of your clavicle is the same as your hip bones, but your waist is also even in width. If you can answer yes to four or more of these questions then this is your body type:

- You do not feel that a meal is complete without dairy products.
- You enjoy cereal and milk if you cannot think of what else to eat.
- You suffer from ongoing fatigue.
- You enjoy dairy products but recognize milk intolerance or have been told you are lactose intolerant.
- You have the same body size as when you were a teen. Your shape may be described as boyish, wiry, or having baby fat, but it has remained the same into maturity.
- You matured later in life and are the youngest looking member in your family.
- You may have an on-going bowel problem (constipation to diarrhea) including spastic colon.
- You have soft fat all over the body, not just held in one area.
- You do not make your mind up quickly and need to have all the information possible to make a decision.
- You are considered to be smart or a nerd in school.
- Your body shape tends to be straight up and down. If a woman you have to use a belt to recognize a waist.
- Your head may be large to your body.
- You consider yourself sensitive to foods or pills.

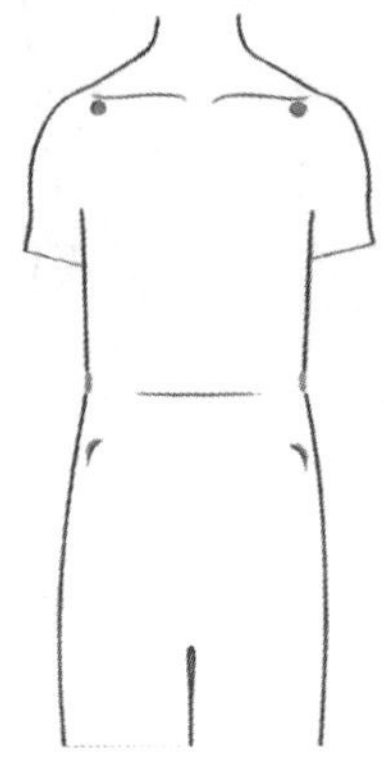

People may see themselves in more than one category. However, all of us are more suited to one category than others. This category is known as our primary or driving biochemical type. If you feel you are several types, you may find you are out of balance. The more out of balance we are, the more we think we are several types. When in balance, you will be the stronger of your primary type.

WHAT YOUR BIOCHEMICAL TYPE TELLS YOU ABOUT HEALTH AND DIET

You may have already concluded that the foods you crave are the very ones that cause many of your problems. The reason for this makes a great deal of sense. We all want to eat foods we enjoy; foods we were given as children. Many times our bodies are still requiring certain necessary nutrients that we cannot sufficiently get from foods that we do not properly digest. As we grow older, our ability to produce the necessary enzymes to digest our favorites decreases. Many of us are born with certain enzyme deficiencies. Poor eating habits developed in childhood, along with stress, only compound the problem. My clinical experience demonstrates that when depleted or deficient enzymes are restored through supplementation, the body comes back into a healthier balance, and a balanced body heals itself.

When a client enters my office, my staff has become very proficient at recognizing what enzymes are lacking to break down particular foods just from observing the client's body type. Furthermore, the staff can correctly anticipate how the client will fill out the questionnaire. You do not have to have Ph.D. written after your name half a dozen times to see the link between enzymes and body types. We all need plenty of naturally occurring enzymes for proper digestion. By giving our bodies the insufficient or missing enzymes for digestion, along with proteases taken between meals for assisting the body to rid itself of toxins, we make for a healthy digestive system. A healthy digestive system thereby can utilize its own enzymes along with the supplementation to break down foods and unlock access to their nutrients.

Our biochemical type determines which foods will create digestive difficulties or weight imbalance. It is thus good for us to take a closer look at the genetic programming that dictates our shape, size, and food cravings. Each person has a genetically programmed ideal weight. If we are overweight, we can still remember when we felt and looked our best.

Biochemical Type One craves sugars or those foods that form glucose (sugar) in the system. It is easy for you to want to be a vegetarian if you are this type, because you will many times only desire starch and sugar. Starch foods are those carbohydrates derived from grains. Some of these are: rice, wheat, potatoes, pasta, bread, and cereals. Vegetables and fruits are carbohydrates as well, and break down into sugar or glucose. Most foods contain trace amount of carbohydrates (sugars). These include granulated sugar, maple sugar, honey, and molasses. Simple sugar is fructose or fruit sugar. Double sugars are sugar cane, beet sugar, maltose (malt sugar), and lactose (milk sugar). All ripe fruits contain natural sugar. Enzymes critical to the breakdown of these foods are various carbohydrate-splitting types that include different amylases, lactase, cellulase, invertase, pectinase, and maltase. Amylase is an important enzyme if you need help breaking down starch. Body Type One is deficient in all carbohydrate-splitting enzymes of which there are 13 different enzymes, not just amylase. Also because of the genetically modified foods, this type may suffer from gluten intolerance and require a formula specific for this problem.

Food cravings create a vicious circle. The more exhausted a Type One feels, the more he or she will crave carbohydrates and starches. They must have their "fix" of sweets, especially chocolate. Chocolate has a huge following of addicts because it is a blend of over 500 flavors. It stimulates the taste buds more than almost any other food. Its melting point is just below the temperature of the human body, so the texture and sensation of it melting in our mouths have great appeal. Chocolate is a perfect combination of 50 percent fat and 50 percent sugar, so it can stimulate certain brain chemicals with perfect equanimity. One of these is serotonin, a chemical that fosters calmness and mood stability. The other, of course, is those famous endorphins; those chemicals that send our "feel good" messages to the brain. Endorphins give us a high level of energy and a feeling of euphoria. When our serotonin level is depressed, we crave potatoes, pasta, bread, and other sugar foods.

Body Type One has been found to be low in serotonin. This absence is usually inherited. We make 99 percent of our serotonin molecules in our digestive tract alone.

I do not recommend that you go cold turkey and stop eating problematic foods overnight. First, it is very important to learn why these cravings exist. The next step is to control them so that the harm they are causing ceases. This is where supplemental carbohydrate-splitting enzymes work wonders. If you make the choice to eat your toxic or foods that cause imbalance, then be prepared to supply your body with the enzymes that will offset or properly digest them. A Type One will always find a way to get a "fix" of the food he or she craves. Now, with supplemental enzymes there is a way to control these cravings.

Carbohydrates and starch foods that are improperly digested cannot be used to feed the brain. Instead, they ferment in the system creating every problem starting from inflammation to fatigue. This type is susceptible to thyroid problems, colon cancer, hypoglycemia, and nervous disorders such as depression and/or anxiety. The main reason for their thyroid problems is the deficiency of hormone thyroxin derived from protein, as these types tend to be drawn to other foods that do not assist the thyroid.

Biochemical Type Twos tend to be attracted to wine if they drink alcohol and foods that are starchy, fatty, flavored, or salted. For example an Italian meal including foods like bread, pasta, pizza, Caesar salad, and wine usually does it for them. This is the case unless you already recognize you do not feel good from eating these foods and they irritate your gallbladder. Fatty and rich foods stimulate the gonadal system (the sexual organs), which creates a feeling of control and high energy. As with other imbalances, these feelings only last for a short while. The craved foods for this type wreak havoc with the gallbladder. I do not need to spend very much time on fat facts. The media has made our entire nation very aware of the harm that man-made fats can cause. The extent to which we have stayed away from good fat and the more adverse health conditions have come into play. For instance, today we have children as young as two years of age suffering from cholesterol problems. I have been called in to assist with newborn babies with gallbladder issues. Every now and then we have many adults having serious heart problems due to plaque in the arteries, obesity, and kidney and gallbladder stones. The human body needs about 35 to 40 percent of good fat in their food each day, however the Type Two may often consume that amount in the form of bad fat or synthetic fats. Some of the other body types are in danger of not consuming enough healthy fat leading to skin ailments. This does not apply to Type Twos. The skin disorders they suffer are caused by other conditions. They are also attracted to chocolate as Type Ones, but they do not eat it necessarily for the same reasons. Type Twos love the blended fat in the chocolate and what it does for their sex hormones.

Characteristic bloating, water retention, and early constipation compromise the Type Two immune system. These body types produce a lot of mucus and suffer more constipation early in life than any of the other groups. They often go from constipation to diarrhea and thus they do not even realize they are constipated. These are the types who will come to my office and laugh when I ask how many bowel movements they have in a 24-hour period. They truly have no comprehension of what I am asking. I explain to them that a healthy system will have a bowel movement following each meal, and a minimum of two per day. I find that a Type Two may go for a whole week before there is any movement at all. This can be followed by several days of nausea and diarrhea. When the diarrhea stops, several days more of constipation may elapse. These sufferers are in dire need of lipase enzymes. Lipase plant-based enzymes break down fat during digestion, and when taken between meals it cleanses the system of poorly digested fat. The lipases I use in my formulas do not even require bile since so many of these types have already had their gallbladder removed. If fats are not digested properly, they turn rancid in the intestinal tract. This body type is prone to diabetes, hormonal problems, and skin conditions.

Biochemical Type Three prefers protein to other foods. Like the others, this type enjoys some fat in chocolate or marbled fat in meat. However, they get most of their biochemical cravings satisfied with protein. They tend to answer to meat and potato-raised. Type Threes have greater muscle mass. However, their consumption of excess protein may create problems with their kidneys and liver. If these two vital organs are not working properly, they suffer. Our system has four detoxification centers that are considered major, so it behooves us to take good care of them. One of these is the colon. Remember that if protein is left undigested in the intestines it putrefies. This type has gas most of the time. The other three are the lungs, skin, and kidneys which primary function is to rid the body of excess protein toxins. I have concluded that psoriasis is a condition caused by poor protein and fat digestion. Type Threes require less protein than any of the other types to maintain their muscular structure and yet a poor ability to break down proteins. Through many years of experience, I have discovered that when any body type ingests the enzyme in which he or she is the most deficient, almost immediate relief from bloating and water retention occurs. Protease, the protein-splitting enzyme, is the major digestive enzyme most lacking in Type Three. This body type has a tendency to create hypertension, heart disease, constipation, and lower back problems.

Type Three does like to "feel" things or to stimulate their body. They like alcohol and other stimulants that in time burn out their adrenals. Feeling the fatigue, they look for other ways to stimulate. If they give up smoking or alcohol stimulation, they head towards sugar. They can make the better semi-vegetarians, but usually will not consider it.

Biochemical Type Four is given the food most craved right from birth. These are the people who gravitate toward dairy products. If they were fortunate enough to be breastfed by their mothers, their potential for handling other foods is greatly improved. Most Type Four people with health problems were not fed their mothers' milk. Often, the mothers were unable to provide enough milk or chose to buy formula. This seems to be a sad situation, but more than likely the mothers themselves were Type Four and suffered extreme food allergies. Type Fours will drink milk until told they are allergic or lactose intolerant. Extreme lactase deficiency characterizes this group. In addition, they need lipase plant-based enzymes to break down the fats found in milk products plus protease for the casein protein in the milk product. I have seen firsthand the frustration of these body types. They go to many different doctors in vain attempting to find out why they are sick or exhausted all the time, but they never find satisfactory answers. A tendency to mature more slowly than other types keep Type Four high school boys from being developed enough to be successful in sports. The girls will also not reach puberty as quickly as the others. Later in life they look younger than their peers and keep the same body shape they had in high school. If they gain weight while young, their soft flesh is more like baby fat. They almost always have similar bodies as adults. The other extreme is a boyish, wiry body in both males and females. It is difficult for this type to build muscle and have to work harder than most to do so.

Type Four has additional digestive problems, which make them feel they are sensitive. Their food choices are limited because meat protein generally has no appeal. These body types can have slight to very severe colon problems because of an inability to digest most foods. To counteract the stress put on the colon, they are encouraged to eat more fiber. This makes matters worse as fiber is made up of cellulose and the human body is incapable of producing its own cellulase, an enzyme that breaks down cellulose. When foods containing cellulase are processed, the cellulase so desperately needed to break down the fiber is destroyed. Another vicious circle is created. Luckily, if given the proper formulation of enzymes, digestion becomes much more efficient. The skin begins to clear and the hair glows with a healthy sheen.

When we feel ill, most of us seek the services of an allopathic physician. Allopathic, as opposed to naturopathy, is a method of medical practice that treats symptoms. Within this framework, a patient is treated with remedies that produce the opposite effect of those created by a disease. Under the care of these doctors, who are responsible medical personnel, we often feel better for a time. However, in many instances, the symptoms return again and again. Unfortunately most medicines are enzyme inhibitors, which force our bodies to work harder than necessary to fight off infections and diseases.

Unsatisfied, we turn our attention toward the alternative healthcare community, exemplified by health food stores, nutritionists, and dietitians. By now we may be experiencing rapid weight gain or loss, constant lethargy, or exhaustion; a mountain of debt from all our expenses towers over us, and we become angry. I am sure at least part of the following nightmare has something to offer that relates to your own personal experience.

Have you experienced this? Someone has just told you that eggs are bad for you. You blink, because you had scrambled eggs and hash browns cooked in grease, along with fried bacon or sausage, served every single Sunday morning while you were growing up. No; now it's okay to eat eggs again, after you've struggled to give them up. Eggs have good cholesterol as it turns out. In fact, we know that the whole egg is to be eaten rather than just the egg white because synergistically they need each other to work as the highest protein. Protein is important; no, don't eat protein! Eat according to the food pyramid and you'll be fine. No wait, that's all wrong, but here, I have a new food plate for you to try. Isn't it great? Now we have genetically altered foods, the wave of the future, say the scientists. But you ask, are they dangerous? The government is not required by law to tell us whether a food item has been genetically altered. The topsoil blew away years ago—but be sure to eat agricultural products. Never eat dairy, it causes too many allergies. Fast and you will cure all your ailments. Don't fast, your body will begin to consume itself. Eat margarine instead of butter. Now we have conclusive proof synthetic fats are much worse than natural ones. Be sure to read those labels in the supermarket. Never mind that the small amounts of toxins added to our food do not have to be reported. Are you confused, frustrated or angry yet?

In the following chapters you will find out how knowledge of your body type can lead to a state of optimum health. I will answer many questions about this critically important topic. You will understand why you hold fat where you do, what foods give your body type energy and what foods create fatigue, why we all have food cravings, why you react differently from another body type to the same food item, how your emotions are affected by biochemical type... the best time for you to eat... why you gain weight... what enzymes you need... why you feel brain fatigue or anxiety... why you suffer nausea from certain foods... and a host of other points worthy of consideration.

Chapter 3

A Personalized Plan for Each of the Types

BIOCHEMICAL TYPE ONE

A typical Type One is born with specific characteristics such as body shape, food cravings, and personality traits. If you are a Type One, you are aware of the powerful energy and drive that you feel when you are stable and secure. You are very intuitive and highly thought of for your wit and caring attitude towards others. When in a healthy balanced state, you are very much in control of your world. When out of balance, you typically experience cold hands and feet, skin problems, hypoglycemia, and fatigue. You may even feel cranky when your glucose is quickly falling, and you might want sugar to bring yourself back into what you consider a happier mood. You may have an inability to utilize B vitamins, vitamin C or properly absorb calcium. Your primary enzyme deficiencies are carbohydrate-splitting enzymes and, over time, you may develop a shortage of protein spilling enzymes (proteases) as well. This chapter will provide a list of energy-producing foods for your body type.

You may be surprised to see that some of your favorites are not listed. The missing items represent foods that do not help you to create balance in your body type. For instance, carrots are rich in sugar. Unless they are cooked, they can create gastrointestinal distress in your stomach. Some vegetables may require steaming if you must eat them. It is preferable to simply avoid the items that are not listed for balance. All fruits should be raw and ripe. Fruit juices are usually high in sugar for you. Bananas have high sugar content and gastrointestinal distress may follow depending on your body type.

FOODS FOR TYPE ONE

VEGETABLES (should be eaten in a raw state or steamed whenever possible):

Broccoli	Cucumber	Peas
Brussels Sprouts	Green Beans	Sprouts
Cabbage	Leafy Greens	Sweet Peppers
Cauliflower	Mushrooms	Zucchini

REDUCE OR AVOID: or take extra supplemental enzymes when consuming

LEGUMES:

Asparagus	Celery	Okra
Beets	Carrots	Eggplant
Garlic	Peppers	Onions
Radishes	Spinach	Tomatoes
Potatoes	Sweet Potatoes	

Avoid: Soy products such as Tofu, Mung beans, and Chickpeas (Garbanzos)

FRUITS:

Apples	Grapes	Pears
Avocados	Lemons	Pineapple
Cherries	Mangos	Plums
Figs	Melons	Prunes
Grapefruit	Oranges	

Eat Fruit raw and be sure to take enzymes when ingesting

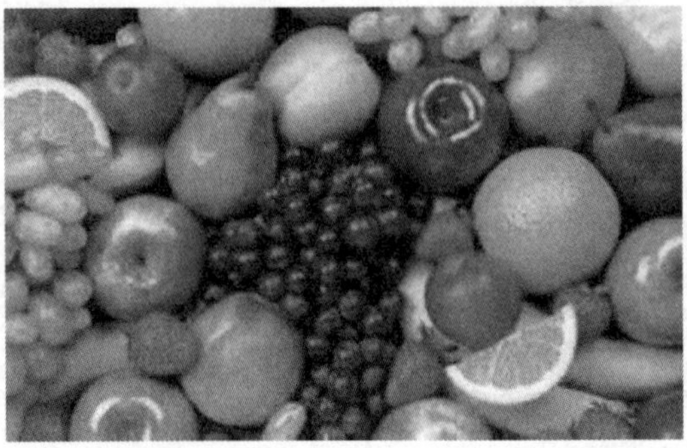

GRAINS:

Barley	Oats	Wheat
Brown Rice (if not gluten sensitive)		

DAIRY:

May have Cheese (white and soft) but all Organic Yogurts (plain)

NUTS:

Sunflower Seeds	Almonds	Most kinds of Nuts

NOTE: Nuts should always be roasted to remove the enzyme inhibitors. Peanuts are the most difficult to digest.

OILS:

Olive Oil or Coconut Oil is best for you

PROTEINS:

Fish	Poultry	Eggs
Beef	Lamb	Game Meats
Seafood		

NOTE: Complete proteins or Brown Rice and Black Beans eaten at the same meal, and proteins are not stored in the body.

FOODS TO AVOID:

Coffee	Synthetic Sugars	Refined Sugars
Sodas	Simulating Drinks	Red Bull or Monster Drinks
Desserts	Fruit Juices	Fried Foods
Heavy Oils	Refined Grains (white flour)	

NOTE: If you have had problems in the past with some of the foods listed here, supplemental enzymes will greatly assist your digestion.

BIOCHEMICAL TYPE ONE HEALTHY CHOICES

Breakfast: Eggs (organic or no hormones fed) or choice of plant proteins, one piece of raw fruit, and raspberry tea. Start your day with more proteins than carbohydrates. If you want bread, make sure you are not gluten intolerant. If not, eat complex carbohydrate bread such as seven-grain, or nut breads rich in proteins. It is very important to start your day with proteins. A good suggestion would be a healthy protein drink that has at least 25 grams of protein. You also use organic raw sugars instead of synthetic sugars. Take your digestive enzymes with 8 oz. water.

Lunch: Large green salad with choice of poultry or fresh fish, brown rice, and raspberry tea. Take one piece of raw fruit for dessert. Eat only raw organic fruit (one selection). Take digestive enzymes with 8 oz. water.

Dinner: Choice of organic chicken, turkey, fish or beef that is grass fed, raw salad and/or steamed vegetables. Limit your starchy vegetables such as white potatoes, sweet potatoes, and most breads. Take digestive enzymes with 8 oz. water.

ENZYME THERAPY: TYPE ONE

Every time you eat, be sure and ingest multiple digestive formulations containing high carbohydrate-splitting enzymes, 7500 FIP lipase enzymes, or 75,000 HUT Protease. You should take enough digestive enzymes to match the amount of food eaten. For example, the meals I have suggested may require two to three capsules per meal, depending on the strength of the formulation and your own digestive health.

The best protease formulation should include at least 375,000 to 400,000 HUT (units of protease) to cleanse and fortify the liver and blood. Take these in-between the meals. Your health may require you to take several capsules per day. During menopause you may need one capsule with meals.

An enzyme formulation with healthy glandular organs would be good for you to support your endocrine system such as thyroid and adrenal. This is beneficial if you have hypoglycemia. These can be taken first thing in the AM and during the day, if required.

A Probiotic (mixed bacterium) formula to balance the healthy bacteria in your large and small intestines would be ideal, since your biochemical type has a weakness for fungal forms and toxicity. Make sure it does not contain a prebiotic FOS since it will cause gas for your type.

BIOCHEMICAL TYPE TWO

You were born with specific characteristics including the way you are shaped, your food cravings, some personality traits—all these added together equal you as a unique human being. When you are feeling well, you are very self-assured, full of enthusiasm and creativity. You are naturally a manager and sensitive to others' needs. When you are in a state of balance, you have great confidence in your world and yourself. Type Two learns very quickly. You use your wonderful imagination to make the world a better place for everyone. When you are out of balance, the health problems you are most likely to experience are allergies, indigestion, gallbladder issues, arthritis, skin conditions, and weak kidneys. A male of this type must be careful of your prostate health. You are deficient in lipase and may be unable to utilize fatty acids, make healthy sexual hormones, and have problems with fat soluble vitamins (vitamin E, D, K omega acids). The list on the following page suggests energy-producing foods for your body type. If you tend to skip breakfast and only drink coffee, then around 11 a.m. you finally eat something—this is very counterproductive to your good health.

ENERGY-PRODUCING FOODS FOR BODY TYPE TWO

VEGETABLES (should be eaten in a raw state whenever possible):

Asparagus	Garlic	Onions
Beets	Green Beans	Radishes
Carrots	Okra	Turnips
Cucumber		

Steam the following vegetables:

Broccoli	Eggplant	Potatoes
Cabbage	Mushrooms	Tomatoes
Cauliflower	Peas	Zucchini
Celery		

LEGUMES:

Mung Beans	Kidney Beans	Chickpeas
Red Lentils		

FRUIT:

Apricots	Grapefruit	Oranges
Bananas	Grapes	Papaya
Berries	Lemons	Cherries
Mangos	Plums	Dates
Nectarines	Tangerines	Figs
Pineapple		

GRAINS:

Oats	Rice	Wheat

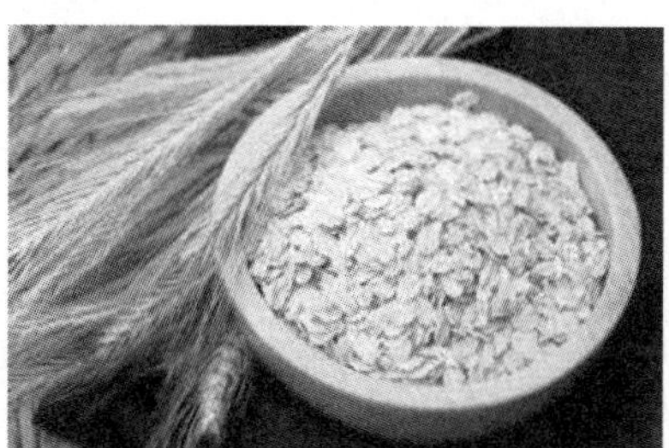

DAIRY:

Yogurt	Cottage Cheese	White & Soft Cheeses

NOTE: No low fat because it is high in sugar. It is best to eat the foods from nature rather than man made foods. Your body can at least recognize "real" food. Real butter is healthier than the man-made chemical butters.

NUTS:

Pumpkin Seeds	Sunflower Seeds	Walnuts

OILS:

Olive	Safflower	Sesame

PROTEIN:

Chicken Breast	Blue Fish	Red Snapper
Cornish Hen	Cod	Sword Fish
Skinless Duck	Halibut	Snapper
White Fish	Salmon	Lean Meats
Turkey Breast	Rainbow Trout	Sole
White & Yellow Perch	Striped Bass	

NOTE: Without hormones and or from the wild

AVOID: Scavengers (Lobster, Shrimp & Oysters), Albacore and Anchovy. All fried food.

FOODS TO AVOID:

Spices	Creams	Organ Meats
Margarine	Rich Desserts	Pork
Bad Fats	Ice Cream	Fried Foods

NOTE: All synthetic sugar as it will create imbalanced hormones

NOTES:

(1) Eat apples sparingly, they may cause gallbladder discomfort.

(2) Increase digestive enzymes when eating dairy products. These items produce mucus and allergies without the proper enzyme action.

(3) Nuts are acceptable in small servings. Be certain they are good quality and take a digestive enzyme with them.

(4) Always use spices in moderation. Minimize or avoid dill, saffron, turmeric, parsley, and coriander seed.

(5) Take your digestive enzyme supplement with all foods.

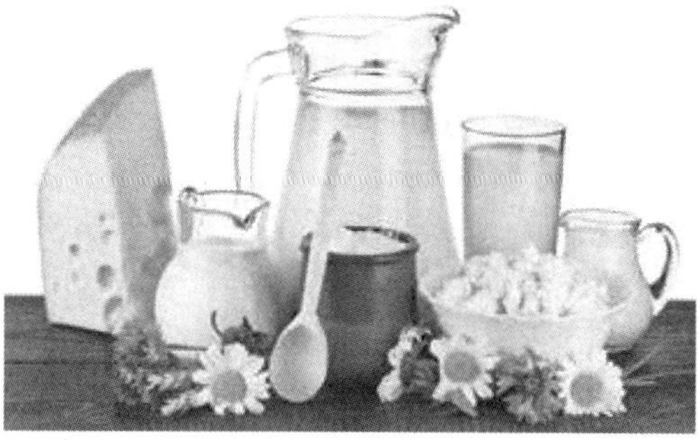

BIOCHEMICAL TYPE TWO HEALTHY CHOICES

Breakfast: Take fruit from your list, organic yogurt, or scrambled eggs/ omelet with vegetables, and herbal tea. It is important for you to break fast by eating breakfast. You will feel healthier if your lunch meal is the largest meal of your day and the dinner meal is your lightest. If you just drink a cup of coffee without food it may set your gallbladder off early in the day. Take digestive enzyme formulation high in lipase enzymes with 8 oz. water with each meal.

Lunch: Green salad or vegetables, organic fowl, organic cottage cheese, eggs, or plant protein. One raw organic fruit selected from your list. Take digestive enzymes with 8 oz. water.

Dinner: Choice of organic chicken, turkey, or fresh fish, brown rice and raw fruit for dessert. Take digestive enzymes with 8 oz. water.

NOTE: Fats and spices may over stimulate your gallbladder. If you have skin problems, they can be controlled with these choices for your type.

TYPE TWO: ENZYME THERAPY

Use multiple digestive formulations high in at least 75000 FIP or more of lipase, with ample amounts of the other digestive enzymes in each capsule. The food that adds weight to your type is starch. Your digestive enzyme formula must have a good number of carbohydrate-splitting enzymes. Take them according to the size of the meal you will eat. If you are bloated or have indigestion, take the capsules immediately before and directly after the meal. In addition, you should take lipase between meals for imbalanced cholesterol or triglycerides. A high dosage of 400,000 HUT protease should be taken between meals to build the immune system and assist with cholesterol (lipo-proteins). Before going to bed, it is advisable to take a probiotic bacterium product preferably containing *L. Plantarum* for good colon health.

BIOCHEMICAL TYPE THREE

You are born with traits that are unique to your body type, just as the other biochemical types. Your inherent body shape, food cravings, and personality are examples of these characteristics. When you feel you are in control of yourself and your world, you have immense power and drive. You are very perceptive. When you are in a state of balance, you can be a leader in whatever you choose. The common disorders you suffer when you are out of balance are exhaustion, body aches, high blood pressure, constipation, and insomnia.

With this type, the body fails to properly utilize synthetic vitamin C (ascorbic acid), amino acids, and properly absorb Calcium/Magnesium. The main enzyme deficiency is protease. Lack of protease enzymes, which break down proteins, may lead to kidney stress and a buildup of uric acid. This can further result in gout, kidney stones, and water retention.

A sense of bloating or flatulence is common to this body type. You can go fairly easy without meals or breakfast until you begin to eat later in the day leading to over-eating (consume more than you can efficiently break down in one meal). You will find yourself eating a lot of food during supper without stopping up to your bedtime.

It is necessary for you to properly understand protein foods. Digestion of protein takes place mostly in your stomach. A small amount of plant proteins is digested in the small intestines where proteolytic enzymes hydrolyze proteins into their constituent amino acids. Your enzymes then enable these amino acids to pass through the walls of your intestine and into the rest of your body. Trillions of your body cells pick up these amino acids and then rebuild them into molecules for new cells and tissues.

For your body type, proper assimilation of proteins can be a problem. These undigested proteins are consumed by microorganisms (bacteria in your system), thus forming gases. These bacteria's use the undigested protein, and release ammonia gas as a result. The liver will now be bombarded with toxins, which will also affect the kidneys. Your lymphatic system, which also works to remove toxins, will suffer. Therefore, it is essential for you to take your supplemental plant-based enzyme formula with your meals, which includes strong blends of protease enzymes.

ENERGY-PRODUCING FOODS FOR BODY TYPE THREE

VEGETABLES (should be eaten raw whenever possible):

Asparagus	Celery	Onions
Beets	Eggplant	Peas
Brussel's Sprouts	Radishes	Garlic
Peppers	Cabbage	Leafy Greens
Carrots	Mushrooms	Cauliflower

NOTE: Sweet Potatoes, Zucchini, and Carrots are to be used sparingly. Tomatoes should be cooked. This is unless you eat organic or homegrown tomatoes.

LEGUMES:

Eat Kidney Beans in moderation.

NOTE: All are acceptable except Tofu. Tofu is from soybeans, which contain estrogens and your body type may convert these estrogens into improper hormones and increase your likelihood of breast problems. Men will have enlarged breast and women may develop breast cancer. Right now the soybeans in the US are genetically modified.

FRUITS:

Apples	Cranberries	Pears
Apricots	Pomegranates	Cranberries
Avocados	Grapefruit	Grapes
Mangos	Melons	Oranges
Papaya	Pineapple	Plums

NOTE: Be careful of very juicy fruits like grapefruit or other Citrus Fruits. They create bloating for this type.

GRAINS:

Barley	Corn Rye	Millet
Buckwheat		

Hot cereals and steamed grains are too moist and heavy for you to begin your day. They will create a bloated feeling unless taken with enzymes.

DAIRY: Organic only

Milk	Yogurt	Cottage cheese

NOTE: Always choose the lower fat dairy products. They are difficult for you to digest without enzymes.

NUTS:

Sunflower Seeds	Pumpkin Seeds	Walnuts

Note: Reduce your intake or completely avoid these nuts. Protein is difficult for you to digest.

SPICES:

Use salt sparingly, particularly if you are accustomed to using it in every meal. You tend to want to salt everything, even melons and some fruit.

OIL:

Safflower	Canola	Olive
Sesame		

PROTEIN:

Poultry	Beef – grass fed	Fresh caught or wild Fish
Eggs		

FOODS TO AVOID:

Salty Foods	Salt	Red Meat
Pork	Organ Meats	White Flour
Fried Foods	Heavy Oils	

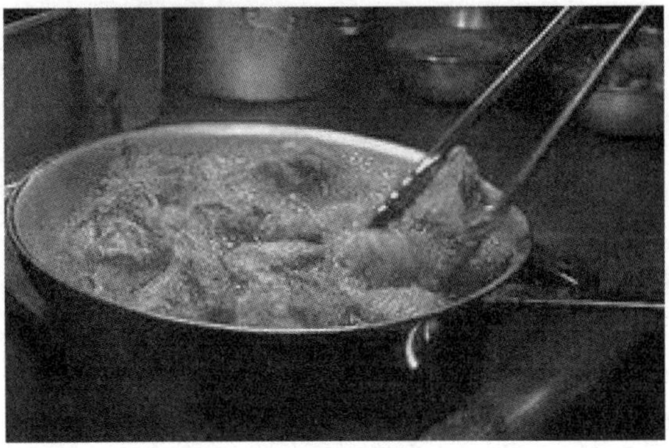

NOTE: (1) Do not eat without digestive enzyme supplementation. This is not just because of your imbalanced cholesterol, but also because of your overall difficulty in digesting proteins.

A semi-vegetarian diet is ideal for most of you. If some of these foods have been troublesome for you in the past, plant based digestive enzymes will help you with digestion. That should be sufficient to take care of any problem you may have suffered with from bloating, gassy, or burps.

TYPE THREE HEALTHY CHOICES

Breakfast: Light organic cereal or seven-grain toast, raw fruits, decaf coffee, or herb tea. Your breakfast should be light compared to the other types. You digest your proteins easier in the evening and this may be the reason why you tend to neglect breakfast. Take supplemental digestive enzymes with 8 oz. water.

Lunch: Large organic green salad, with fish and fruit. Do not use a creamy-style salad dressing. You may prefer a vegetable protein rather than fish. Take supplemental digestive enzymes with 8 oz. water.

Dinner: Choice of organic chicken, turkey, or fresh fish along with steamed or raw vegetables and raw fruit. This is the meal at which you will have the easiest time digesting your protein. If you choose beef, make sure it is grass-fed without hormones. Take supplemental digestive enzymes with 8 oz. water.

ENZYME THERAPY: BODY TYPE THREE

Take multiple digestive formulations containing at least 70,000 to 110,000 HUT of protease activity, plus appropriate amounts of multi-enzymes in each capsule. The dosage should reflect the quantity of food you are eating. This also depends on the strength of the formulation, especially the protease enzyme.

You need a systemic protease enzyme formulation, which must contain at least 400,000 units of protease activity to fortify the liver and blood. Protease is the enzyme that is most important for your body type. Take this regimen several times per day between meals. When you are over 50 years old, you may want to take a capsule of protease along with your supplemental multi-enzyme formula with meals.

A multi Probiotic (bacterium) product is vital to keep the pH and healthy bacteria constant in the small and large intestines. I suggest they should be taken before bed for your type. This helps prevent further gastrointestinal problems.

As we age, we become less efficient with our metabolic enzymes and begin having problems breaking down proteins. This is even more important for you and my suggestion is that, if you are over 50 years old, you may need to introduce more protein and double the amount of protease when you eat it.

BIOCHEMICAL TYPE FOUR

You are born with specific traits such as your body shape, your food cravings, and the assorted qualities of your personality.

When you are enjoying a state of good health and stability, your mind is very clear and creative. You tend to be a reflective, logical thinker and visionary. As long as you maintain balance, you are in complete control of your world and you overflow with helpful information for others. You may have been known as a nerd in high school because of the quality of your intelligence.

You are out-of-balance when you have these symptoms; allergies, milk intolerance, aching knees, gas, fatigue, nervousness, skin breakouts, and irritable bowels. The common enzyme deficiencies that occur in your body type are lipase and carbohydrate-splitting enzymes, especially lactase. This means that your needs are more difficult and complex than those of the other body types. In this case, you possess an inability to assimilate fatty acids, amino acids, and fibrous natural foods. The list on the following page includes the energy-producing foods best suited for your body type.

ENERGY-PRODUCING FOODS FOR BODY TYPE FOUR

VEGETABLES: Although the other three types do better with raw vegetables, you should steam yours. This is why some of you suffer from indigestion and gas after eating salads. I am aware you may have heard that steaming kills the enzyme action in these vegetables, and therefore it would seem better to eat them in a raw state. Remember, these types of enzymes are made dormant in the human stomach and thus unable to assist in the digestive process of the small intestine.

Tolerating raw foods can be difficult because your digestive system is very sensitive.

VEGETABLES:

Asparagus	Green Beans	Onions
Cauliflower	Leafy Greens	Peas
Celery	Mushrooms	Spinach
Eggplant	Okra	Tomatoes
Garlic		

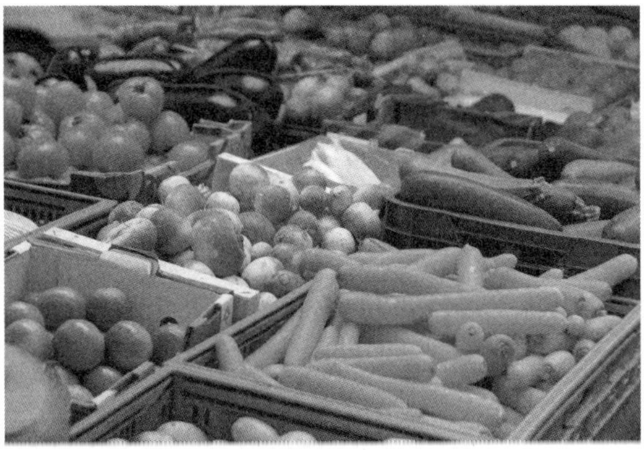

VEGETABLES to avoid or reduce amounts consumed:

Beets	Carrots	Sweet Potatoes
Broccoli	Cabbage	Cucumbers
Zucchini		

NOTE: Take extra digestive enzyme supplements when consuming

LEGUMES:

Mung Beans	Lima Beans	Garbanzos
Kidney Beans		

FRUIT:

Apples	Figs	Plums
Grapes	Lemons	Tangerines
Grapefruit		

NOTE: Fruit must be very ripe and eaten raw. Avoid canned or frozen fruits.

GRAINS:

Buckwheat	Barley	Toasted Grains
Brown Rice	Oats	

DAIRY:

NOTE: Dairy products act as a stimulant to Type Four and should be taken sparingly. They are the most difficult for you to digest and they create mucous and allergies. If you eat them, be sure to take supplemental digestive enzymes with lactase enzymes.

PROTEIN:

Poultry	Beef	Fish—wild
Eggs		

NOTE: Beef should be organic or grass fed. Protein is most important for your body type. You have always needed protein foods but have preferred to get them in dairy. All complete protein is necessary for your type for muscle and healing.

NUTS:

Almonds	Coconuts	Cashews

NOTE: Most nuts are okay if roasted or sprouted.

OILS:

Virgin Olive Oil	Sesame	Coconut Oil

FOODS TO AVOID:

Ice Cream	Sour Cream	Fried Foods
Cheese	White Flour	Sugar
Margarine		

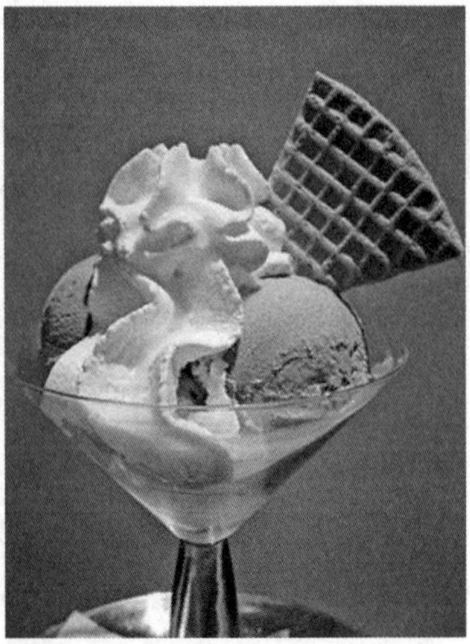

NOTE: You should also remember to take supplemental enzymes when you consume any dairy products.

NOTES: Protein (casein) and sugar (lactose) from dairy sources are your big problem areas. Therefore, a good alternative for you would be fish, poultry, and eggs. It is very important that you obtain amino acids in food form since they are building blocks. Spices should be used cautiously. Please remember, these are not the only foods you can eat, but they are the best ones for keeping your biochemical type in balance. Supplemental digestive enzymes are a necessity for your sensitive digestive process.

BODY TYPE FOUR HEALTHY FOOD CHOICES

Breakfast: Have a substantial meal with protein. It is extremely important for you to begin your day with protein. Have this with some raw fruit. Be careful with cereal and milk; they throw you out of balance, although you may like them at every meal. Take supplemental digestive enzymes with 8 oz. water.

Lunch: Choice of organic poultry, fish or eggs, steamed vegetables, and one piece of ripe fruit. Take supplemental digestive enzymes with 8 oz. water.

Dinner: Choose another protein from your list, more steamed vegetables, a whole-grain roll, herbal tea, and raw fruit for dessert. Take supplemental digestive enzymes with 8 oz. water.

TYPE FOUR ENZYME THERAPY

Take multiple plant-based digestive formula containing at least all the carbohydrate-splitting enzymes high in lactase. If you eat dairy, you will need additional lactase at 8,000 ALU.

You need a systemic protease enzyme formula that contains at least 400,000 units of protease activity to fortify the liver and blood. Take this regimen several times per day between meals.

A bacterium product taken at bedtime should help prevent irritable bowel syndrome. I suggest multiple probiotic for sensitives, which do not include sugar-based prebiotics.

If you are overweight or have any other condition related to enzyme deficiency, you might want to look at the Renewal Program.

Chapter 4

What Biochemical Gut Type Are You?

Research out as of April 18, 2011 classified humans into categories of bacterial ecosystems. This came as no surprise since I've believed for many years that we are all part of distinct or separate biochemical systems and what works for one does not mean it can work for all. You probably have heard the phrase "different strokes for different folks." It is exciting to recognize these truths in accordance with the research.

WE ARE NOT ALONE!

This research refers to enterotypes (bacterial system in the human gut) after collecting poop samples from around the world, which classify people into three categories of microbes. One of the three possible types of the DNA we carry around, is about 1 percent human and the other DNA belong to the 10 x 100 trillion cells in microbes (bacteria) that hang out in our gut. We are not alone—we coexist with our gut microbes! The estimated 10 x 100 trillion individual bacteria live in our intestines, making up the complex ecosystem that is the gut microbes. These bacteria help to break down food (produce their own enzymes), protect us against attacks by pathogens (80 percent of the immune system is in the gut), and play a vital role in health and nutrition (produce enzymes to make some amino acids, minerals, and vitamins) in our colon.

ANOTHER ORGAN!

In a recent interview with Professor Tine Rask Licht, an expert in gut health and the winner of the 2010 Danisco Award for her research in the field, said that recently there has been a shift towards starting to consider the gut microbes as an organ in itself. Since we coexist with these microbes, this relationship can become pathological as in obesity, diabetes, arthrosclerosis, and inflammatory bowel disease. Change of diet is the best way to control these mutants.

These ecosystems are named Bacteroides known as Enterotype 1, Prevotella recognized as Enterotype 2, and Ruminococcus referred to as Enterotype 3 microbes (bacteria), which do produce conditions that are different from each other. You might think that this depends on where we live, what we eat, our nationalities and other variables, but actually, you would be incorrect. It is what you host, as defined in the beginning of your life, and what your organisms entertain or invite to their lively gathering from the food that you consume through life.

A newborn is born without these bacteria, but hopefully the baby is breastfed and the mother's breast milk contains microorganisms that balance microorganisms. However, everyone else who handles the baby shares his or her microorganisms. Your mother's and father's health at the time you were conceived, plus the way you handle your proteins, will define your type. It is all about diet controlling the good or bad bacteria.

Enterotype 1 - Bacteroides ecosystem has high levels of gut bacteria and enjoys fermenting sugar from the starch you eat and proteins which produce enzymes to make vitamins C, B2, B5 and H.

Enterotype 2 - Prevotella ecosystem has fewer bactoids and likes to dine on mucosa proteins from the lining of the gut. These showed higher producing numbers have B1 and folic acid-producing flora.

Enterotype 3 - Ruminococcus ecosystem happens to be the most common. They also like to dine on gut mucous proteins, but they also really enjoy sugar treats. They produce biotin, riboflavin, pyridoxine, and vitamin B12.

This new biochemical ecosystem information fits nicely into the Biochemical typing I've taught for years. The different types recognize the body's ability or inability to properly break down food and feed the body's ecosystem (bacterial community).

WHICH GUT TYPE ARE YOU?

Are you taking the correct probiotic strains? The proper strains are those that will feed each other and not neglect one or more of the three base strains the research mentions.

Sadly, the numbers of the biochemical types and the enterotypes do not match from when I first named my types by numbers. *Try not to get confused.* See the following paragraph.

- Type One – thyroid/parathyroid – carbohydrates problems = Enterotype 3
- Type Two – hormonal/gonad – fats & starch problems = Enterotype 1
- Type Three – adrenal/suprarenal – protein problems = Enterotype 2
- Type Four – pituitary/nerve – dairy & starch problems = Enterotype 1

YOU ARE WHAT YOU EAT

I have always stated that we are what we ingest. If we cannot break down our foods properly, we will become toxic. The type of food we eat and digest, or fail to digest, make up the three enterotypes I just wrote about. The research published in science found that intake of meat, fat, carbohydrates, and alcohol appear to influence the type of bacteria that thrive in the gut. However, the study also suggests that dietary changes may not mean we can quickly replace one microbial population with another.

PROBIOTICS SEND SIGNALS FROM YOUR GUT TO YOUR SKIN

Much more is known about how probiotics work in your gut than what is known about their effects elsewhere in your body. However, new research shows that there may be signals coming from these gut microorganisms that are sent to your skin and mucosa. It seems that probiotic benefits are not limited to your digestive system. These gut microorganisms are sent throughout the body and interact with your skin and gut mucosa. This is exciting news since they hope to improve skin conditions such as dry skin or irritations.

At first, this may seem strange to you that they could play a role in your skin health, but when you consider your skin is bathed in bacteria, it does not seem such a stretch after all. We know there are about 100 trillion cells in the body and ten times the number of bacteria, fungi, and more living in and on your body. Bacteria living within and on you form a symbiotic relationship. Think of your body as its own living ecosystem, teeming with beneficial bacteria and enzymes keeping you alive!

I have pictures of children with eczema treated with enzymes and probiotics that clear in a matter of weeks. Breastfeeding mothers who take supplemental digestive enzymes and probiotics protect their infants from skin disorders, respiratory problems, and various diseases. If a mother does not breastfeed, then she should give the infant appropriate probiotics for protection against diseases for an additional eight months.

PERSONALIZED PROBIOTICS

A similar approach as nutrigenomlcs (personalized nutrition) indicates that research might also be applied to probiotics, wrote Prof Kleerebezem and his co-workers, anticipating that a person's response to probiotics may not only be determined by the probiotic strain consumed, but also the person's genetics, their diet and lifestyle, and their 'resident macrobiotic.'

"This study could be among the first steps to investigate the interplay between macrobiotics, probiotics, or other nutritional supplements and human genetics to personalized nutrition," they added.

CONCERN ABOUT USING THE RIGHT STRAINS

There has been a five-year study in Japan, which led to improvement of probiotics. It was established early on that the majority of the lactic acid bacteria would lose their fight or are killed before they made it to the large intestine. I began using probiotics at the very beginning of their introduction and have kept them refrigerated making sure they were living strains. Just recently, I have been interested in a prebiotic that is not a sugar base. I have only used one kind of prebiotic, and that is artichoke heart that controls the amount of good bacteria. Prebiotics have been sugar based and genetically modified. By that, I mean they will assist the good and bad bacteria to multiply. There has been no control over the strain they assist.

The study recommends products that contain several strains of naturally developed organic acids that are encapsulated along with important strains of lactic acid bacteria, vitamins, minerals, and amino acids. This is what I've been formulating for years. It is wonderful that I now have research to back up my theory. You need to be assured that the strains work together and do not destroy each other. When the strains are proper, the amounts that the body can deal with our immune system does not have to come into play and attack those it does not recognize as an invader.

There is now confusion between the importance of supplemental digestive enzymes compared to probiotic supplementation. The confusion has been common enough that we have received emails from doctors asking which one is the most important. They each have different duties in the human body. Grant you, the probiotic can manifest its own protease enzyme in the large intestine to assist in removal of toxins, but they do not do the necessary work in the cell that enzymes do. They are both necessary for health but have diverse functions.

BIOFILMS—WHAT ARE THEY?

A Biofilm begins with the attachment of free-floating microorganisms (bacteria) on a surface. Similar to slime bacteria we know of as in "slime in the ice machine." Another way to describe it is a biofilm is like a tiny city in which microbial cells, each only a micrometer or two long, form towers that can be hundreds of micrometers high. The "streets" between the towers are really fluid-filled channels that bring in nutrients, oxygen, and other necessities for live biofilm communities.

Some Biofilm require a grouping of microorganisms housed in a matrix (held together) made up of primarily polysaccharides and proteins. The organisms produce these for their protection. In a healthy GI tract, the biofilm is a thin layer containing beneficial bacteria that support digestion, nutrient exchange, and provide immunity functions. In an unhealthy GI tract, the biofilm becomes thick and hosts pathogenic organisms that become very resistant to antibiotics and antimicrobial treatments and may contribute to a myriad of illnesses.

BIOFILMS AND INFECTIOUS DISEASES

Biofilms have been found to be involved in a wide variety of microbial infections in the body. And by one estimate, 80 percent of all infections involve biofilms. Infectious processes in which biofilms have been implicated include common problems such as urinary tract infections, catheter infections, middle-ear infections, formation of dental plaque, gingivitis, coating contact lenses, and less common but more lethal processes such as endocarditis, infections in cystic fibrosis, and infections of permanent indwelling devices such as joint prostheses and heart valves. More recently it has been noted that bacterial biofilms may impair cutaneous wound healing and reduce topical antibacterial efficiency in healing or treating infected skin wounds. It has recently been shown that biofilms are present on the removed tissue of 80 percent of patients undergoing surgery for chronic sinusitis. In other words, they can grow anywhere, including in the human body.

Bacteria growing in a biofilm are highly resistant to antibiotics, up to 1,000 times more resistant than the same bacteria not growing in a biofilm. Standard antibiotic therapy is often useless, and the only recourse may be to remove the contaminated problem. You may have heard of Salmonella, Streptococcus, or E. coli strains because of food biofilm. Since the biofilms are all around us, and in some cases in us, I began looking for the appropriate probiotics and in this case, a prebiotic to go with it. I absolutely could not use the prebiotics which are sugar derived because they do nothing to balance out the biofilm. I am thrilled to say I finally found the proper prebiotic and probiotics to fight off the strains of Salmonella, E. colis, and Streptococcus in biofilms. This is an added problem when traveling and developing Montezuma's Revenge. I recently formulated it, and there are several cruise lines and airlines interested in the product. It would be wonderful if before you left on a trip you could begin the product, and take it during your trip so you can enjoy yourself without worrying if you will spend most of your trip in your room's bathroom and miss out.

Probiotics are very important because we are never alone in this human body of ours!

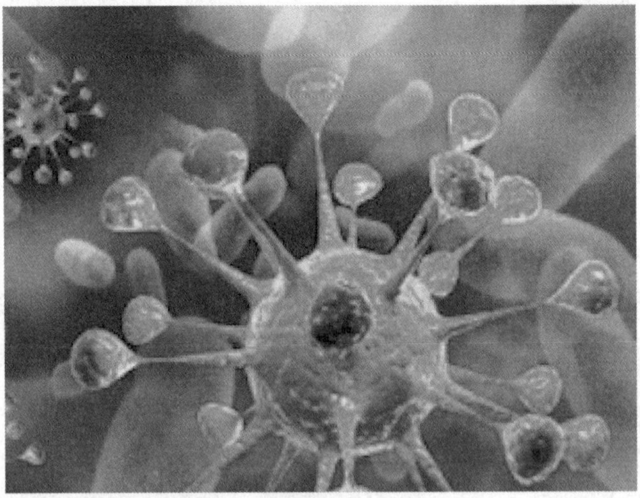

TESTIMONIALS

"Thank you so much for allowing me to be part of your research on TravelZyme. The first thing I noticed was the size of my stomach began to go down within the first day. My trip went without one problem with the food I ate. I take your digestive product and protease, but what a wonderful thing to have no worries when on my trip in a country where I generally have immediate problems with diarrhea. It has ruined my trips more than I can tell you. God Bless You!" - Sarah H. - Denver, CO

"Dr. DicQie I appreciate all you have done for me on my health journey. Once we got me on the appropriate probiotics for my type, I no longer face constipation or gaseous outbreaks. I took probiotics for years, but now I understand why they did not work for me like others. My life is so much more joyous!" - Cara C. - Las Vegas, NV

"My doctor loves our probiotic. He has many missionary families on it. And now I am getting the story 3rd generation about how all the 'others' got 'travelers' disease, and the ones who were taking your probiotic did not get sick." - D Aubrey - Austin, TX

Chapter 5

New Life For Your Digestive System

WHAT IS WRONG WITH MY DIGESTION, AND WHY CAN'T I EAT THE FOODS I USED TO EAT?

Many people have been asking the above questions to health-care practitioners throughout the last few centuries without getting an appropriate answer or solution to their problems. It is completely wrong to say that the body can easily digest and assimilate food. This has been the thought of many people in the past as well as today...Consumed food passes through the digestive tract more slowly than you think. Therefore, it tends to ferment and putrefy, "throwing toxins" into the system. These cause gas, heartburn, headaches, eye problems, allergies, and a host of other serious conditions.

Supplemental plant-based digestive enzymes are used in the gastrointestinal tract with a purpose of breaking down food. Under optimum conditions, this process accomplishes three things: (1) it digests food; (2) nutrients are absorbed into the cell; and (3) waste products pass through and are eliminated. Supplemental plant-based enzymes are much more beneficial than animal enzymes because they are activated more quickly in the digestive system. They begin their work immediately after ingesting, while food is still in the upper part of the stomach.

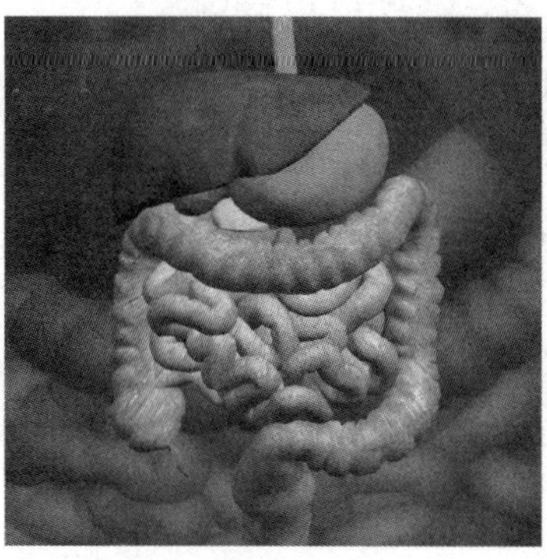

Sometimes, they are activated while dissolving in the esophagus. We all know papaya and pineapple as sources of enzymes that break down protein. They require a pH that is not commonly required by the stomach. Rather, it is aspergillus plants (single-cell plants), which are grown on natural foods, that are the most worthwhile source of digestive enzymes. They perform more efficiently in humans, insuring the digestion of fats and carbohydrates as well as proteins. Aspergillus enzymes serve a dual purpose: They prevent waste from entry and storage in our cells, and cleanse cells of old waste matter. Your digestion is only as efficient as your stomach's ability to begin the process.

For you to be healthy, your system has to assimilate food, distribute the nutrients, and eliminate waste through the bowels. All these should happen without any discomfort or gastrointestinal stress. Earlier, we learned that carbohydrates can ferment, fats turn rancid, and proteins putrefy. This undigested material is known as food remnants. A major problem with undigested food is that it often passes into various parts of the body to place where it is deposited as waste. This problem manifests itself as high cholesterol, calcium deposits, arthritis, cellulite, and more seriously, as plaque in the arteries.

Let us now review once again what it is that supplemental digestive plant enzymes do:

- Protease enzymes: break down proteins
- Lipase enzymes: break down fats
- Amylase: breaks down starch
- Cellulase: breaks down cellulose (roughage)
- Lactases: break down milk sugars
- Sucrase: breaks down sucrose (refined sugar)
- Invertase: breaks down simple sugars
- Alpha-galactosidase: breaks down legumes
- Beta-glucanase: breaks down cereals
- Glucoamylase: breaks down rice and other starch
- Hemicellulase: breaks down vegetables
- Macerase: breaks down fiber in fruit
- Pectinase: breaks down the skins of fruit
- Phytase: breaks down fiber in vegetables and grains
- Xylanase: breaks down fiber wall of plants

It is good to understand that our bodies do not manufacture cellulose—we must ingest it. In addition to digesting fiber, cellulase transforms into cellulose and glucose and short-chain fatty acids. With food allergies becoming a common problem and more genetically altered foods appearing on the market, we must make enzymes a part of every meal. The other listing of carbohydrate-splitting enzymes our bodies do not produce either. Eating raw does not mean we properly break down many parts of the vegetable or fruit as we once thought. Many nutrients are found in this roughage.

NOTE: More detailed information on enzymes at the end of this chapter.

GALLBLADDER

Burping, belching, a bloated feeling, hiccups, intestinal gas, regurgitation, discomfort in the rib cage area, nausea, diarrhea, breathing difficulty, overall exhaustion, heartburn, anxiety, rapid heartbeat, headaches, and constipation are the results of a stressed gallbladder. Lumped together, we describe them as "indigestion." Gallbladder problems are triggered by the body's inability to break down fats because of excessive alkaline or excessive acid pH in the digestive system. If you have any of the following symptoms, you may have gallbladder stress or disorder:

- Nausea or diarrhea after eating, immediately or hours later
- Headache before or after eating
- Nausea relieved by eating or a bowel movement
- Burps and belches
- Fatigue after eating
- Indigestion
- Diarrhea followed closely by constipation
- Pain or tenderness in the right upper abdominal area
- Bloating or tenderness at the base of the sternum (breastbone)

Poor eating habits cause stress in the gallbladder. More bile is produced when too many man-made fatty foods are ingested. This causes peristalsis; hence, the occurrence of nausea or diarrhea is more probable. Some of the irritating foods to the gallbladder include apples, a few raw vegetables, some grains, fruit juices, Brazil nuts, and all seeds. Fatty and highly-seasoned foods such as ice cream and most other desserts, Mexican, Italian, and Chinese cuisines, and chocolate may also irritate the gallbladder if bile is insufficient or you have a buildup of hardened bile.

TYPES OF GALLBLADDER IN RELATION TO INDIVIDUAL BIOCHEMICAL (BODY) TYPE

In Type One, gallbladder stress occurs through overeating of rich carbohydrates. Type Two suffers similarly but adds to this—poor fat digestion. If a low-protein and a high-carbohydrate diet are followed, then insufficient bile is produced. If this happens, the gallbladder cannot empty itself, and the liver is not stimulated to produce the correct amount of bile. This leads to fats remaining in large particles. Hence, incomplete fat digestion and absorption. The undigested fat combines with any iron or calcium contained in the food to form insoluble soaps, which prevent minerals from reaching the cells. These hard soaps can cause constipation, anemia, and bone loss. In addition, the lack of bile acids also prevents the absorption of carotene, Vitamins A, D, K, and essential fatty acids. This leads to a multitude of deficient disorders. By now, you are beginning to understand why eating healthy food only is not enough. Lack of proper digestion of food or inappropriate foods for your body type, may cause many problems. This leads to one of the serious problems called continued depression of the immune system. This is where multi-enzyme supplements can be very effective.

HIATAL HERNIA

Hiatal hernia is a weakened, stretched, or protruded muscle forcing the stomach through a hole in the diaphragm. This interferes with the production of hydrochloric acid because the vagus nerve is pinched, causing discomfort and pain since food cannot enter the stomach and leads to undigested food particles being exposed to bile. Bile, which is an alkaline substance, acts as a strong soap. The delicate balance of chemicals is disrupted, and the bile washes away the protective coating of mucus in the stomach that guards against extremes of acidity and alkalinity. The cells 'work overtime' to produce extra hydrochloric acid to counteract the excess alkaline bile. The area then unprotected by the mucous coating becomes an irritated lesion, or ulcer. If this happens to the stomach, where good digestion must begin, the entire digestive process is undermined. Some of the difficulties you might encounter with hiatal hernia include belching, bloating, intestinal gas, regurgitation (a burning sensation which feels as if the food has not gone all the way down), discomfort underneath the rib cage, nausea, diarrhea, constipation, difficulty with breathing, exhaustion, pressure and pain in the left side of the chest, anxiety, rapid heartbeat, and headache! Often, patients in emergency rooms think they are having a heart attack when the real condition is gastric distress or hiatal hernia. There is a small dissimilarity between gallbladder and hiatal hernia symptoms because they are closely connected. A hiatal problem is first triggered by poor fat digestion, which puts undue stress on the gallbladder. Likewise, gallbladder problems can be the result of a hiatal hernia, depending on what types of foods ingested, and whether disruption of the acid/alkaline balance takes place. Later in this chapter, I will discuss the importance of good acid and alkaline balance.

What is wrong with my digestion? The best answer to this question is the supplemental digestive enzymes. Research has shown that a combination of the proper enzymes restores pH balance throughout the digestive tract. In the case of the hiatal hernia, if supplements are taken with the meal, the enzymatic action could begin even in the protrusion. Introduced enzymes would stabilize the balance between alkaline and acid stressor food types.

FOOD ALLERGIES

Food allergies should really be named food sensitivities, which are nothing more than the body's toxic reaction to substances that it cannot break down. The word allergy means an abnormal and individual hypersensitivity to substances that are ordinarily harmless. Numerous case histories show positive results from the use of digestive enzymes as a treatment for food allergies. Eighty percent of our immune systems are in our digestive tract. Common sense shows when we supplement with enzymes, we can boost a digestive process that has ceased to produce enough enzymes or signals for enzymes on its own. When we do this, our food allergies disappear. Because we as different people have different biochemical types, we will differ in the amount of time, number, and variety of enzymes we will need to be able to reintroduce safely irritant foods into our diets.

As an example, I will discuss the importance of good digestion, which begins with the pancreas. The pancreas produces enzymes for digestive action. If the pancreas has undergone too much stress from overuse through improper eating, it becomes overwhelmed. It can no longer meet the excessive demands placed on it. Upon the pancreas losing its ability to produce pancreatic proteolytic enzymes, an insufficient quantity of various enzymes is created. One consequence is poor digestion of proteins into amino acids. The amino acids make up proteolytic enzymes. And if amino acids are deficient, these enzymes, which prevent and eradicate inflammation, will be ineffective. This sets off a chain reaction that reduces enzyme production elsewhere in the body.

Other areas adversely affected by these deficiencies are hormonal activity; excessive demands for vitamins, mineral, and trace minerals; lowering of immune defenses; infection; and a general feeling of malaise. The end result is unusable protein molecules that are intended to fight inflammation. Instead, they are absorbed through the intestinal mucosa and circulated in the blood, entering tissue in partially digested form. These partially digested protein molecules are known as peptides. The body regards them as invaders since they cause a kinin-mediated inflammation. Kinin chemicals cause pain upon contact with nerve endings or tissues of specific organs. Nature has charged the pancreas with the essential task of providing enzymes to control inflammation, regardless of its cause. It could be due to a cut, a bruise, or a chemical reaction in the food we ingest.

Conventional medicine has produced chemically based anti-inflammatory drugs that reduce inflammation. However, these drugs do not cure chronic inflammation. It matters greatly to our overall health what foods we eat, or whether we smoke or drink, because this has much to do with our own nutritional state. If we are unable to break down our food into small enough particles, we will suffer from inflammation of the organs as well as the joints. This can manifest as edema or tissue swelling, histamine, sinus and allergy problems, and a general loss of good health. This ultimately leads to dependency on antihistamines, nasal sprays, chemical tranquilizers, antidepressants, and aspirin. Anyone who is nutritionally deficient, infected, toxic, or has food addictions will suffer the same consequences. These develop into chronic degenerative illnesses unless something is done to stop the progression. I firmly believe that enzymes are necessary for the good health of everyone. My clients with chronic illnesses have all been afflicted with poor digestion for a significant number of years. Prevention is the best prescription. Remember, it requires you to stop something before it happens!

GASTRITIS RELIEF

The important enzymes for treating gastrointestinal disorders are large amounts of protease, carbohydrate-splitting enzymes including amylase, lipase, and a small quantity of cellulase. Some herbs may also be helpful as well. I personally recommend Marshmallow Root in the enzyme digestive product. This herb works effectively in assisting the body to manufacture the materials that build new tissue. It has the adhesive property that allows it to surround and expel foreign or toxic matter. Marshmallow Root has a soothing effect on inflamed mucosal membrane tissue in both the gastrointestinal and respiratory tracts. This helps to normalize mucous secretions and remove excess accumulations of uric acid. Another very effective herb is Gotu Kola. It is known as a longevity herb; it is rich in vitamins and minerals. Marshmallow Root used in conjunction with Gotu Kola works even more efficiently. Any discussion of herbal remedies for all kinds of irritation cannot leave out Prickly Ash. Prickly Ash is a powerful treatment for the bowels, lungs, and stomach. Many herbs, when used in correct proportion with the right enzymes, can produce a very calming effect if emotional stress is the cause of your gastritis. One of them is Valerian Root. Others are Hops, Skullcap, and Wild Lettuce. To normalize this crisis, whether emotional or physical, you must continue to ingest the basic enzymes with each meal and then follow with a soothing blend of herbs and enzymes.

ULCERS

The peptic ulcer occurs most commonly. It is defined as the loss of the tissue lining of the lower esophagus, the stomach, or the duodenum. Less serious, but often confused with ulcers, are lesions. They involve the muscular coat but do not constitute a complete loss of it. These lesions are not as painful as ulcers. While many people know that gastric acid and pepsin are partially responsible for ulcer formation, it is unknown why mucosal resistance to them should become impaired. Bacteria are the cause of many ulcers. There are many theories about how genetic makeup and environmental conditions can cause a peptic ulcer. We do know that the symptoms get much worse from eating hot diets and spicy foods. Psychological stress may also alter gastric functions. We know that stress can create ulcers. A stress ulcer differs clinically from a chronic peptic ulcer. It is more acute, but not as painful. Severe trauma or surgery can trigger stress ulcers. Some ulcers are caused by overuse of certain drugs, such as aspirin or alcohol. The symptoms include burning or gnawing pain, cramping, or aching. Medical professionals describe the pain as coming in waves, each of which can last several minutes.

In my experience, ulcers can be treated in a similar way to other gastric problems. Remember, Protease breaks down bacteria that do not belong in the body system, so it would naturally be beneficial for a bacteria-induced ulcer. As described earlier, the same herbs and enzymes used in combination with one another would also prove to be very effective. These herbs and enzymes can actually help to rebuild the mucosal lining. I have formulated a product that aids in the replacement of the mucosal lining over time. This solution includes treating the body with love and care so chronic health problems will not have an opportunity to develop. It is very wise to start your children on enzymes at an early age, rather than waiting until they have contracted an illness of some kind.

DIARRHEA

I find it very interesting to hear what the average person thinks of as normal or natural concerning bowel elimination. When clients call me complaining about diarrhea, I ask them about their symptoms. Is it an explosive, uncomfortable diarrhea? It can also be the kind that can be serious due to the loss of electrolytes. Are you spending a great deal of time on the stool? Alternatively, have your bowels merely changed; are they less thickened or hard? Do you go to the bathroom more often? There is a difference between diarrhea and a loose stool. Diarrhea can be dangerous when the rapid evacuation of fecal matter results in the loss of water and electrolytes and other essential substances, like potassium. This produces an acidosis that creates further problems. Besides frequent bowel movements, there are usually abdominal cramps and an overall weak feeling. Sometimes the stools are coated with blood, or they contain mucus. When we change our diets and eat more raw vegetables and fruits, this creates looser and more frequent stools, a condition not to be confused with diarrhea.

At the onset of diarrhea, take a natural product designed to control it. If it lessens the number of bowel movements and is not very painful, then you know this is not a chronic problem. However, if you cannot get it under control, it is best to see your doctor immediately. Many of my clients, especially Biochemical Type Twos—those drawn to spicy and fatty foods—create an imbalance through the overproduction of bile. When bile is thin or produced frequently, it creates peristalsis (muscle action of the colon). This causes several bowel movements in rapid succession, or diarrhea. A stressed gallbladder can create the same problem, also directly related to the type of foods you eat.

If foods are digested correctly and the body is able to get from them the nutrients it requires, you would never have diarrhea. As our health improves, our stools become more like they were when we were babies or young children; they are rather formless. If you eat two to three meals per day, then you should have two bowel movements per day in order to stay healthy. Some of my clients have actually told me they have diarrhea because they have more than one bowel movement in twenty-four hours! There are those body types that fluctuate between constipation and diarrhea. Poor eating habits can cause an endless cycle of several days of constipation followed by several more of diarrhea. It often becomes very troublesome and persistent. In this case, the results of treating the problem with enzyme supplements have been phenomenal. In most instances, the diarrhea becomes outdated. On the other hand, if the diarrhea is infrequent, it may not be directly caused by what you eat but because you cannot digest correctly. Use of the supportive herbs described in the Gastritis Relief section can bring a calm, balanced effect upon the gastrointestinal system. Lipase is the best enzyme to use for diarrhea control, as it works in "harmony" with the gallbladder. In addition, it breaks down fats. Incomplete fat digestion may lead to diarrhea in certain instances. Protease along with lipase will eliminate inflammation that may occur.

CONSTIPATION

My past years of practice as a colonic therapist taught me the importance of a healthy bowel. Colon irrigation confirmed my belief that very few people experience good digestion, assimilation, utilization, and elimination.

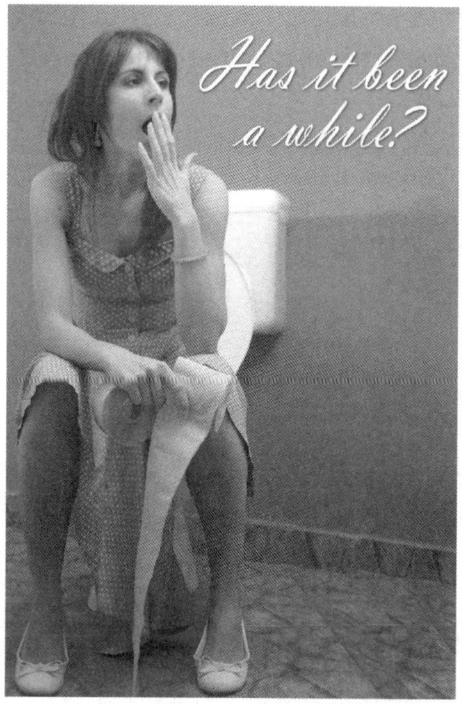

When digestion improves, so does the elimination. Elimination is every bit as important as digestion and assimilation. Toxemia, the outcome of accumulated and un-expelled feces and other waste matter in the body, is a dangerous and inevitable effect of constipation. A clean and clear colon is vital to our good health. Few of us recognize that failure to effectively eliminate waste products causes a tremendous amount of fermentation and putrefaction in the colon. Neglect of this accumulated debris can, and frequently does, result in degenerative diseases.

If you eat processed, fried and cooked foods, starches, sugar, and excessive amounts of salt, your colon cannot possibly stay clear. Even if you have the requisite two or three daily bowel movements, it remains clogged with old waste. These foods, instead of nourishing the muscles, tissue, nerves, and cells of the colon walls, actually starve it. A starved colon may let a good deal of fecal matter pass through it, but it is unable to activate the final stages of digestion and nourishment for which it is intended.

When the mineral elements that compose the foods we eat are saturated with oil or grease, the digestive organs cease to process them efficiently. They are passed out of the small intestine into the colon in the form of debris. In addition, the body disposes of a great deal of used cell and tissue matter in the colon. As these undigested waste materials pass through the system without assimilation, they leave a coating of slime on the inner walls of the colon, like plaster on a wall. With the passage of time, the coating will gradually increase in thickness until there is only a narrow opening in the center. The matter to be evacuated contains much undigested food from which the body can derive little or no benefit. Sickness at any age is the direct result of loading up the body with foods that have no vitality; that are not digestible. Allowing the intestines to remain "crowded" with hard waste matter is further cause of illness.

THE COLON—YOUR BODY'S SEWAGE DISPOSAL PLANT

The colon is a natural breeding ground for bacteria, of which there are two types. These are the healthy, scavenging type such as bacilli coli, and the pathogenic or disease-producing kind. Healthy bacteria in the colon neutralize, dissipate, and prevent toxicity from developing. When too much fermentation and putrefaction occur, the pathogenic bacteria proliferate and ailments result. A normal colon is equipped with a very efficient elimination system. In simple words, the colon is the sewage system of the body. If we do not keep it as healthy and free of disease as possible, our major organs and glands are seriously compromised. The colon affects every one of the body's organs. It is intimately related to every cell in the body. The primary purpose of the colon is as an organ of elimination. It collects all terminative and putrefactive toxic waste from every part of the anatomy. Through peristalsis, the contraction of the colon muscles, all solid and semi-solid waste is removed. The best of diets can be no better than the worst if the sewage system is crowded with a collection of waste. It is impossible, when we eat two or three meals a day, not to have a buildup of residue in the form of undigested food particles, as well as the end-product of digested food. On top of everything else going through the colon, the body has to rid itself of the toxins or waste products, including our millions of cells that have served their purpose.

Remember, the colon plays an extremely important role in the final stages of digesting food and energizing all systems of the body. The residue coming from the small intestine (chyme) still contains some uncollected nutritional matter. The colon is supposed to extract this matter. It mulches this matter and then transfers the liquid and other elements through its walls and into the blood stream. The blood carries it to the liver for processing. Obviously, if the feces in the colon have putrefied and fermented, any nutrients present would pass into the blood as polluted products. This is a condition known as urea. This substance can be measured through a urine test to determine the level of toxicity of the body. Lumen of the colon contains intestinal flora for lubrication. Fecal encrustation interferes with the infusion of this flora. It also causes a severe lessening in the peristaltic action needed for evacuation. Further, the ability to absorb and use the additional nutrients present in the waste residue that enters from the small intestine is badly compromised. A human bowel can extend to five times its normal size. Imagine the quantity of accumulated, packed feces that can be stored in an unhealthy colon! All this fecal matter in the bowel only serves to intensify a state of constipation. Anyone who eats three meals per day but experiences less than two bowel movements in that same period is in a constipated state. It is a natural function of our bodies to eliminate waste after digestion.

Constipation is self-poisoning—brought on by lifestyle, stress, too many sugars, and poorly digested food. Autointoxication (poisoning by toxic substances generated within the body) begins with an inability to digest food. This in turn creates toxic fecal matter that remains in the colon. These toxins soon begin to be reabsorbed into the bloodstream. *(See Appendix I for more information.)* The body rids itself of wastes in four natural ways: the colon, kidneys, lungs, and skin are the four major organs of elimination. The bowel produces up to 36 different toxins to be released later into the body system. These toxins affect every cell in our bodies. To assist with elimination, enzymes are absolutely necessary. For those who suffer from chronic constipation, there are enzymes that should be taken after meals and before bed. Others can restore vital, healthy bacteria in the large intestine. These bacterium-fortified enzymes act as a natural antibiotic in the intestinal tract. Most overweight people are constipated.

Normally, digestive enzyme formulations are taken at the beginning of meals so that they arrive in the stomach at the same time as our food. I have heard some people say they have no problems with digesting any kind of food, yet they may have difficulty with regular elimination. I believe people say these things because they are not well-informed. It is the purpose of this book to educate you about the importance of enzymes. Only then can you make wise choices for proper maintenance of your health.

Chapter 6

What's Making Me Sick, and What Do I Do About It?

ACID / ALKALINE BALANCE

Our bodies naturally seek a point of balance in all our systems, and the process of digestion is one of the most important ones. Good digestion will affect your breathing, elimination, nervous system, blood pressure, insulin / sugar controls, and hormones, among other functions. The body works continuously, 24 hours a day, to maintain the proper acid/alkaline balance in the body. This process is known as homeostasis. If this balance is not well maintained, the metabolic enzymes and all other biochemical activity will not function normally. Acid-producing medications, drinks, and some foods—the greatest of which is sugar—bring on acidosis. The body's two buffering systems, the lungs and kidneys, can control it. These systems control the fluids composed of sodium, protein, and phosphate. The vagus nerve, running throughout the entire body, plays a vital role in good health. If it is pinched by a hiatal hernia, then it reduces the acid level.

When food is prevented from entering the stomach because of hiatal hernia, it is not broken down to the extent it should be because hydrochloric acid was not released. When food comes from the stomach and reaches the duodenum, bile alkalinity is produced. This acts as an abrasive soap that washes away the mucous coating that the stomach uses to protect itself from extremes of alkalinity or acidity. The results are putrefaction or fermentation of food, rather than digestion. Hydrochloric acid is the only acid beneficial to the body and is necessary to digest proteins. I do not recommend taking this acid in synthetic form, because I believe it is important for the body to manufacture its own. Protease enzymes assist in that process. If your pH balance is abnormal, you will be forced to breathe very quickly, to counteract the acid imbalance. Because the vagus nerve runs near the heart, the pulse and blood pressure increase. Added to this, the stomach becomes irritated and spastic. The liver and gallbladder overproduce bile, further irritating the digestive tract. Then, the pancreas will produce too much insulin, leading to low blood sugar. Within the small intestine, a reduction in alkaline occurs, causing the whole system to become excessively acid. The large intestine responds with either diarrhea or constipation!

Conversely, too many antacids and diuretics, leading to potassium depletion, bring on alkalosis. In a situation of excess alkaline, the pineal gland overcompensates by producing too much hydrochloric acid. As in all things in the natural world, a perfect order of balance is always maintained. That is called homeostasis, and it applies to our digestive system as much as it does to the path of our galaxy through space. What starts this domino effect of distress? Most people become upset about something in their lives at least several times a day. Are you aware that your stomach contracts at even the smallest negative feeling? Recall some times when you have heard bad news and it felt as if you had been hit in your stomach, or you grab your stomach. Feelings lead to biochemical changes in the body. Emotional difficulties trigger these as much as biological ones do.

We know that when the body cannot get the fuel it needs to run itself efficiently, it will look to itself for life-sustaining chemicals. For example, when it needs calcium and cannot get it because of poor diet, it will take calcium from its own bone. It can break down the white blood cells for enzymes or protein from our own muscle—whatever it takes to remain alive. Added to this, the endocrine glands, your body's mind, become sluggish. These glands are crucial to good health; they control the immune and nervous systems. Without the endocrines functioning properly, imbalances occur in our glucose levels, brain food, and hormones. We can experience erratic premenstrual syndrome, bowel problems, fatigue, and a depressed immune system. Enough has been said about imbalance in digestion.

What can I do to prevent this from occurring? If it already has, what do I do? Laboratory tests and the Biological Terrain Assessment™ using blood, urine, and saliva have proven repeatedly that plant enzymes support correct pH balance. I have taught and used the test to support this. I ask my clients to ingest supplemental digestive enzymes with meals. From a urine specimen, I have observed a constant pH balance of 6.2 to 6.7, with some variation expected due to biochemical type. The optimum pH in urine in 24 hours is 6.4. Doctors who use enzyme therapy have documented the same results thousands of times with various evaluation tools.

We have used Spectra Cell Laboratory, located in my hometown of Houston, which has a method of determining the nutrient needs in the body by using venous blood draw. We did a clinical research with those who take digestive enzyme supplementation and those who do not. The results showed that many supplemental digestive enzyme users did not show a lack of nutrients; and everyone in the group who had never taken the supplements lacked various nutrients dependent on their biochemical types.

CASE HISTORY

A very beautiful young woman, my former client whom I had not seen for several years, recently came to my office. The last time we were together she had just been married and was expecting her first child. She was particularly lovely that day she told me she was pregnant. As the health of her child was very important to her, her OB/GYN doctor sent her to me for advice on diet and enzymes. Throughout her pregnancy and the birth, she carefully followed her enzyme program. However, after the child was born, she became negligent in her daily routine. I have seen this happen so many times. Because she felt better and had the baby, she did not think she needed the enzymes anymore and stopped taking them. Even though all symptoms are removed if you stick with the daily regimen of enzymes, you still need to continue your program. This young woman enjoyed good health for a while after she stopped using them. Soon, the old habits and cravings for sweets, coffee, and pizza were back. She once again experienced fatigue, skin breakouts, hiatal hernia symptoms, and gallbladder nausea brought on by digestive problems. Her husband lost his job, and she had to return to work, leaving her child in someone else's care. Although I was sympathetic to her plight, I simply suggested that she treat herself with the same love and care she had shown for herself and her baby during her pregnancy. Knowing that she could not change her biochemical type since it is something we bring with us into the world, we worked on an appropriate diet for her type and added enzymes back to her diet. Three days later, she called to cancel her appointment. She was already back in control and knew that she would continue on the path toward good health. She learned that her good health was something she owed to herself and her family. To this day, I am amazed when I see her. She exudes youthfulness and happiness. People compliment her on the beauty of her skin, and they constantly comment on how she looks younger every time they see her! Those of us who are in enzyme nutrition hear this story repeatedly. I cannot say it often enough: Education and supplementation are of extreme importance.

When we understand why we have pain or feel ill, we can make choices and stay in control of our lives. For so many years, we thought that if we had a particular symptom, all we had to do was treat it, make it go away, and then resume our old lifestyle. That is how conventional medicine is practiced. However, when you find a health-maintenance program that works for you, you must commit to follow it for the rest of your life. Instead of treating what you have as a disease, or its symptoms, you increase the love you have for yourself and others. That love must include the gift of good health to you.

HOW TO OVERCOME DAIRY INTOLERANCE

When your body can no longer make the correct amount of enzymes to digest a particular food properly, but that food is still consumed, intolerance for it is created. From then on, we experience an allergy or adverse reaction to it. It is a toxic substance for us. This occurs for people who develop a problem with dairy products. Lactose is the offender contained in dairy. The enzyme lactase breaks down lactose. I have my clients take lactase along with other enzymes. Protease is most important in the digestion of dairy because it has several types of protein in itself such as casein. Lipase must be included because of the fat (lipid) content in dairy products. It is advisable to take a multi-digestive formula rather than a single lactase product.

My advice to those who suffer dairy intolerance, or any other kind of food allergy (sensitivity), is to take the enzyme supplements for at least 21 days before trying to eat the food you are allergic to. It takes that long for the system to make a positive response to the newly introduced enzyme support. Then, be sure to take digestive enzymes each time you consume those products. I strongly encourage you to follow this program before you reintroduce foods with which you have had problems in the past.

Gluten Sensitivities: I presented several slides on lectins while in Europe and told the audiences that the human body does not make all the necessary enzymes to properly break down lectins/glutens, which are found in carbohydrates and are part of our inflammation and disease processes. We have recognized lectins/glutens for more than 100 years.

Why has it now become such a problem? To better understand, we first need to be educated in what they are. Think of lectin / gluten as a protein containing a key that fits a certain type of lock. This lock is a specific type of carbohydrate. All life forms, plant and animal, insect and fungus, have cell membranes that contain carbohydrates, which sit within and project from the membrane. When a lectin/gluten with the right key meets, one of these 'locks' on the gut wall, artery, gland, or organ and 'opens the lock', it disrupts the membrane and damages the cell. This in turn initiates a cascade of immune and autoimmune events leading to cell death. During my presentation, I went on to explain supplemental enzymes formulated for this problem could assist in eliminating the cause.

Being gluten intolerant should not stop you from quality of life. Because it is difficult to test conclusively, many people will be diagnosed based on a wide variety of screenings and observations. The most common symptoms are gastrointestinal problems (or gastrointestinal distress) such as diarrhea, flatulence, gas, and bloating. Other symptoms may include joint pain, fatigue, and headaches. Think about the fact that there can be 250 or more symptoms related to gluten intolerances. In fact, it can manifest itself as Candida.

Is gluten intolerance a wheat allergy? Unbelievably you can have wheat allergies but not have gluten intolerance. Confusing to be sure, but they are two different responses in your body. Gluten intolerances or sensitivities happen slowly over a period and are more nutritional deficient. Symptoms of wheat intolerance will manifest itself as a typical allergy; quickly with a single exposure.

To expose the problem in a broader form, let us find an answer to the question posed earlier in this book. Why is it now such a problem if it has been in our foods for hundreds of years? The answer to the question is simple but with serious consequences. Much of our food has been genetically modified, and in doing so has had lectins transferred from animal, plant, bacteria, human, and virus DNA into our foods to enable them to last longer on the shelf or into the seeds to grow foods quicker in a smaller area. They are called GMO (genetically modified organisms). This has confused our digestive systems and since around 80 percent of our immune system is present in our digestive system, the response is an allergy to these foods simply because the body does not recognize them.

What can one do if he or she is suffering from gluten sensitivities? Now that we have a better understanding of what gluten/lectin, and/or wheat intolerances, are and why we are having such a reaction to them, I want to remind you that they are not just a protein problem but also proteins combined with carbohydrates referred to as glycoproteins in food.

When asked to formulate a supplemental enzyme product for these intolerances, the formula must have specific blended proteases required for gluten/lectins found in food. Proteolytic enzymes are necessary for the proper breakdown of casein and wheat proteins. The formula also needs several, yet different, carbohydrate-splitting enzymes called "polysaccharolytic," which work differently from each other because carbohydrates have many different kinds of linkages. The carbohydrate on gliadin is very complex, consisting of xylose, glucose, galactose, and arabinose, which are all plant sugars. It is typical of plant cell walls, which require hemicellulase, pectin, and lignin, for proper degradation. An additional yet specific probiotic named Bifobacterium Lactis is to block the toxic effects and balance the increased permeability to the gut. This type of formula can be a benefit to those suffering from these intolerances and require gut balance.

Because of this growing problem, I was asked to formulate a product specifically for gluten sensitivities.

I received a question about these allergies and the comment was that enzymes do not work for this problem. Actually, supplemental digestive enzymes are necessary when the human body does not genetically produce the enzymes needed for these confusing modified organisms we now find in our food sources. They absolutely **do work** for this problem if it is the correct formulation.

History of treating gluten intolerance is to remove the foods containing gluten out of the diet; you might ask yourself if this is possible? Avoiding the genetically modified organisms by purchasing organic, or growing your own food, makes sense. Nevertheless, when you travel or eat out, quality of life begins to take a back seat. Those of us suffering from this intolerance benefit by taking the proper supplemental enzymes formulated with the necessary probiotic in order to address these hidden gluten/lectins in foods.

SUGAR INTOLERANCE

I believe that most of America is glucose intolerant. By that I mean we have become very lackadaisical about how much food we eat containing high levels of sugar. Sugar is used as a preservative in most foods. The average person simply is unaware of this fact. It appears in surprising places. Any food that has been processed, canned, or frozen includes sugar. We give our children an amazing amount of sugar without realizing it; we are a nation of sugar addicts. A whopping 92 percent of all foods sold in America are combined with sugar to a greater or lesser degree. It is hidden in most food products on the market. The average American eats 1 cup of sugar every day, or 210 pounds a year! Any label that claims "no fat" or "low fat" has high levels of sugar listed on it. Certain soft drinks intended for young people contain 16 to 18 teaspoons of sugar in 12 ounces of liquid! Cereals sometimes contain more than 60 teaspoons of sugar!

Our glucose balance is the most precious and high-precision balance in the body. The brain needs 140 grams of glucose, or we will get a headache. Added to that, we need an additional 40 grams to make and feed red blood cells. Normal function of the brain and healthy blood cells require 180 grams of glucose per day. Yet, we ingest 1,000 grams of sugar each day. How do our bodies handle the surplus? We produce more insulin, which carries glucose to our cells. Hypoglycemia is the end result of overeating sugar. This happens when the body is forced to make enough glycogen to balance the increased quantities of glucose and insulin in the system.

America is "virtually falling asleep" because of eating so many simple carbohydrates (sugar). Sugar robs the system of nutrients as well as creating an acidic state.

So many children are unable to absorb their lessons in our schools because their brains are blocked by too much sugar. Fatigue is rampant among adults as well. I have concluded that sugar is responsible for most of the colon problems we suffer. Most of us still do not realize that overdoses of sugar have far-reaching effects, causing numerous health complications. Enzymes can make a big difference. Amylase and invertase work well in the breakdown of sugar to glucose and help with gaining control of how much we ingest. I only use small amounts with a diabetic. Protease provides a nontoxic environment. This is one way to start the "cleanup" process. However, each of us must take responsibility for our own consumption of sugar. Remember the fatigue, anxiety, and headaches you have while eating a diet heavy with sugar, and it will assist you in your efforts to control your intake.

TRYING TO KICK THE SUGAR HABITS WITH SYNTHETIC SUGAR

If you are using an artificial sweetener, it is probably because you are trying to avoid the calories while still craving that sweet taste. Sweet cravings are very common and quite understandable when you realize that sugar is as addictive as some hard-core street drugs. Unfortunately, switching to artificial sweeteners will neither reduce these cravings nor increase your satiety. On the contrary, you are likely making matters worse. Your body tends to crave sugary foods when it is lacking proper fuel. Sugar is very quick fuel and can give your body a boost when it is running low. However, using artificial sweeteners will not trick your body into thinking it has had its fill; rather it wants more sweets because it didn't get the energy boost that normally go along with the sweet taste. In fact, this is part of why artificial sweeteners are associated with increased weight gain rather than weight loss. You are simply confusing your body.

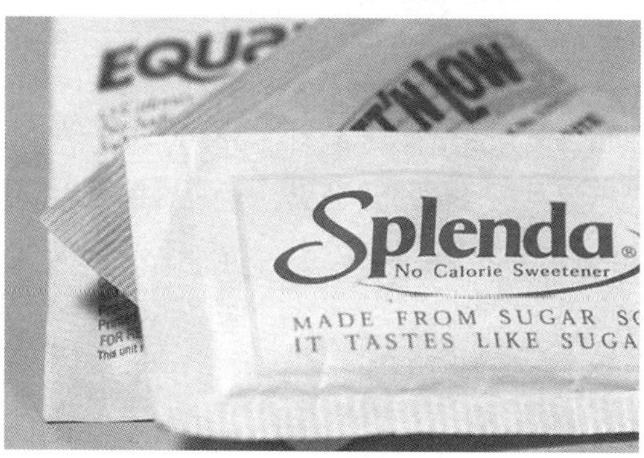

For example, inflammatory bowel disease—an autoimmune disease that can have serious health consequences—may be caused or exacerbated by the regular consumption of the popular artificial sweetener Splenda, as it inactivates digestive enzymes and alters gut barrier function. Previous research also found that sucralose could destroy up to 50 percent of your beneficial gut flora, and increases pH level in your intestines. Many consumers may suffer ill effects from artificial sweeteners such as Splenda without realizing their problems are related to their consumption of artificially sweetened foods and beverages. If you experience any of the above signs and symptoms, you would be well-advised to stop your use of sucralose products.

There really is not a good reason to ingest synthetic sugars. You might be thinking about diabetes and how this is suggested for them. Now science is showing it creates worsening symptoms of diabetes and weight gain.

Since we now know about synthetic sugars, let's talk about other synthetic ingredients...

ARE YOU EATING BEAVER ANAL FLUID WITHOUT EVEN KNOWING IT? (SHOCKING TRUTH!)

Yes, it's true. Millions of people across the globe are eating "beaver anal fluid" and don't even know that they're consuming such a substance.

It's called "castoreum," and it's emitted from the castor sacs within the animal's anus. For a beaver, this slimy brown substance is used to mark its territory, but for us humans, it's used as an additive that is often labeled as "natural flavoring" in the foods we eat—vanilla, strawberry and raspberry being the most common.

Castoreum is a product of the trapping industry. When beavers are skinned for their fur, these glands are taken out and are sold after being smoked or sun-dried to prevent putrefaction.

Why is castoreum used? The most notable characteristic (after being processed) has to be the smell of castoreum. Instead of smelling horrible, like most people would expect from an anal-produced secretion, it has a pleasant scent, which supposedly makes it a perfect candidate for food flavoring and other products.

The question that many people put forth would have to be "who in their right mind actually made this odd discovery?" and reminds me of the common question "who was the first person to eat raw oysters?"

Another industry that uses castoreum is the fragrance world. For decades, perfume manufactures have used it to make various types of fragrances. These anal secretions are said to contain around 24 different molecules, many of which act as natural pheromones to stimulate our senses. From perfumes to air fresheners, beaver castor sacs are quite versatile within the fragrance industry.

IS IT NATURAL?

Sure it's natural, but does "being natural" make it right to use or consume? Many disgusting substances are considered "natural," yet eating them may not be the best idea.

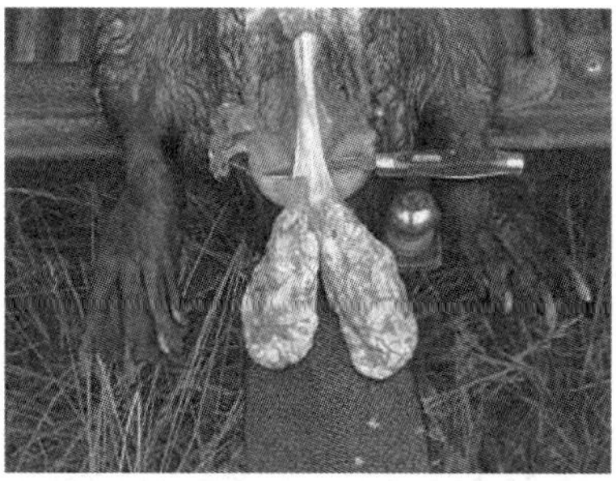

The act of labeling something so vulgar and disgusting as "natural flavoring" should be illegal in many people's eyes, but the FDA views it all in a different light.

Having the anal secretions from a beaver take the place of a strawberry in something like strawberry ice cream hardly seems like an efficient process. Why go through the process of harvesting "anal secretions" when a strawberry is much easier to pick? It hardly seems like a better option...

The food industry is a tricky business to figure out, and it will continue to boggle the minds of many on issues exactly like this. Much like with other additives that have raised concern over the years (aspartame, high fructose corn syrup, and food colorings); castoreum is proving to be just as questionable.

HOW DO I DECIPHER WHAT I'M EATING?

The exact definition of natural flavors from the Code of Federal Regulations is as follows:

> *"The term natural flavor or natural flavoring means the essential oil, oleoresin, essence or extractive, protein hydrolysate, distillate, or any product of roasting, heating, or enzymolysis, which contains the flavoring constituents derived from a spice, fruit or fruit juice, vegetable or vegetable juice, edible yeast, herb, bark, bud, root, leaf or similar plant material, meat, seafood, poultry, eggs, dairy products, or fermentation products thereof, whose significant function in food is flavoring rather than nutritional."*

Whew...Did you get all that? This may be the first time you've ever read that...Now you know why!

When the phrase 'natural flavors' appears on a package, the best move is to call the company and find out what the flavors are actually made from.

Of course, I say this assuming that we're all the kind of people who would be horrified to find out that we might have come close to ingesting fluid from the anal sex glands of beavers.

This certainly is not a product for Vegan, vegetarians, or those concerned about animal rights. The European Beaver was hunted to near extinction, both for fur and for castoreum, which was also believed to have medicinal properties. The North American beaver population was once more than 60 million, but as of 1988 was 6 to 12 million, largely due to extensive hunting and trapping. Although sources report that beaver populations have now recovered to a stable level, some experts say that today's American beaver population is only 5 percent of what it was when Europeans first settled in North America.

Here is a positive if you are one of those people who has stress or need sleep—castoreum in medicine is used for menstrual problems, anxiety, and sleeping disorders.

By the way if you enjoy smoking please understand that castoreum is used for the smell and taste of your cigarettes. Maybe that is where they got the term, "Cigarette butt!"

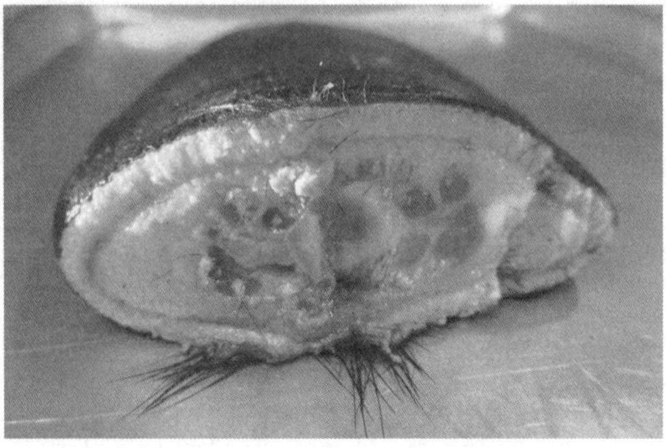

In food, castoreum is used to flavor candies, drinks, and desserts. Read the ingredients on food packages, call customer support when you see those words, **'natural flavors,'** and guess what? You'll never consume anal fluid again.

MONSTER ENERGY DRINKS ARE BETTER BIGGER

Our children and young adults rave about the look of the can and the buzz or rush they receive along with the added excitement of the unknown, maybe a seizure. Forget that their ingredients are a laundry list of huge amounts of:

- Sugars that make up the syrupy goo
- Synthetic sugars that can rattle hormones and add no calories
- Petroleum based artificial colors
- Caffeine anywhere from 80 to 350 mg (espresso has 40 mg)
- Stimulating herbs and brain-blasting amino acids
- Inositol as an effort to keep your body from going into a panic attack
- Whoops, I almost forgot...added synthetic minerals and vitamins

Americans are paying big bucks to feel "energized." We spend nearly $3.5 billion annually on drinks named Rockstar, Red Bull, Power House, Adrenaline Rush, Monster, Spike, and Venom. Eight million adolescents guzzle these beverages on a daily basis, and both casual and dedicated athletes use them to get an extra "push."

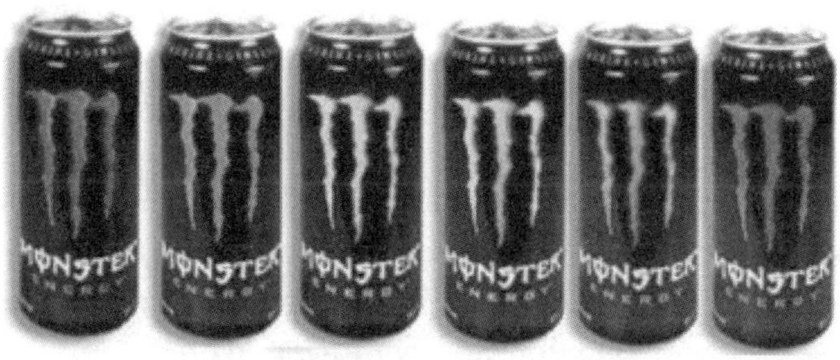

The side effects of energy drinks alone should be enough to discourage you. Some may think they have to take more to get the same "benefits," or may add some alcohol to strengthen the effects. Mixing energy drinks with booze causes further dehydration. This explains why kids are passing out at dance clubs. Energy drink cocktails cause drowsiness, loss of coordination, and slow reflexes. To make matters worse, when you are chugging back energy drinks and alcohol, it's hard to determine just how much booze you've actually taken in. As a result, your blood alcohol concentration will rise together with your energy—therefore you will not even realize how much alcohol you've consumed and might try to do something stupid—like drive a car. There have been many instances with young people dying because of energy drinks and mixing them with alcohol. While mixing some energy drinks with alcohol may taste good, the effects of this could be a fatal mistake. Because there now have been deaths pointing at these types of drinks, they are banned by several other countries.

Moms this paragraph is for you. For pregnant women, experts recommend a maximum daily caffeine dose of 200 mg (many energy drinks contain more). Higher doses increase the risk of miscarriage. Additionally, fetuses can't efficiently metabolize caffeine. The Journal of the American Academy of Pediatrics recently published the concern over energy drink consumption and the youth-aimed marketing. The concern is the interactions, long-term consequences, and dangers associated with risky behavior.

Checking out at the grocery store the other day I found myself behind a very handsome, body buffed, young guy who had only two items in his basket. Hey, I was just looking at his basket! You probably guessed—Red Bull and alcohol. I've started to pay attention to the ages of those I see consuming energy drinks and all this led to investigate websites of the most popular energy drinks. There are hundreds of comments from users on each site stating dying devotions, not caring if they die—they'll die happy—and warnings from some that suffered side effects. This world of toxic dependency on liquid drugs offered in a can to our young people should concern each one of us. European countries are banning the use of energy drinks. Does this mean they care about their children but America doesn't?

Think about America five to 10 years from now. It has always been said that America's strength is their youth. What will a young person drinking these energy drinks today possibly look like as an older adult? Use your imagination on how they might morph into obese, sleep deprived people, suffering heart and blood pressure problems with exhaustion and confusion. Their skin would be wrinkled and aged before their time because of the high dehydration. Wait—is that not what is happening right now?

DIABETES

The medical records of the 19th century are very sparse and incomplete when it comes to any cases resembling diabetes. Why? This is because type II diabetes, or what was formerly known as adult-onset or noninsulin-dependent diabetes, is the direct result of sugar/starch consumption. Refined sugar was not widely used until after Napoleon built sugar factories in Europe in the 19th century. In 1850, the average Englishman consumed only seven-and-a-half pounds of sugar per year. By 2000, we ate 156 pounds. That is how much added sugar Americans consume each year on a per capita basis, according to the U.S. Department of Agriculture (USDA). Imagine it—31 five-pound bags for each of us. They get this by taking the amount of sugar purchased and dividing it up by the total of all Americans. All I can say, someone is getting more than that because our family does not consume sugar unless hidden—which is true for all of us. This year about 25.8 million citizens of the United States have type II diabetes. Some people are born with type I diabetes when from birth, the pancreas is unable to produce the necessary insulin. Type II is characterized by an overabundance of it. Insulin is the pancreatic hormone that regulates the transport of glucose—blood sugar—into the cells. In type II, the body develops a resistance to the action of insulin. When the body fails to respond to insulin, the blood glucose-level rises and pancreatic cells pour out more of the hormone in a vain attempt to process it. Eventually, these cells wear out, causing insulin shortage.

Type II diabetes and its complications affect 25.8 million Americans, costing as much as $174 billion each year. According to the Centers for Disease Control, the number of Americans with Diabetes could triple by 2050. One in 10 U.S. adults has the disease but could grow to 1 in 3 in the next 40 years. Some common occurrences that are suffered by those with diabetes are blindness, kidney failure, and loss of limb. Each year 4.2 million people become legally blind; 202,290 develop kidney failure; and 65,700 lose a leg through amputation. At all ages, people suffering from diabetes have twice the normal death rate.

When we consume large amounts of sugar, the body counteracts with the release of high levels of insulin. Remember, insulin is a hormone secreted by the pancreas. Insulin transports glucose—a form of sugar useful to the body—through the bloodstream and into the cells where it is converted to glycogen. Glycogen is stored carbohydrates. If it is present in excessive amounts, it is further modified into a fat called triglyceride. Copious amounts of insulin contribute to obesity because of this conversion of glucose into triglycerides. When we consume any food that breaks down into sugar, such as fruits, vegetables, or starches, we are taking in a considerable amount of sugar. Even refined carbohydrates eventually break down into glucose, causing your body to overreact. Instead of producing the exact amount of insulin necessary to handle the quantity of sugar ingested, it makes more. This excess insulin is what forces the blood sugar to an even lower level. The consequence of consuming large amounts of sugar causes the body to end up with less blood sugar than it started with, and the result is exhaustion. So what do we do? We eat more sugar for that so-called "mid-afternoon pick-me-up." The body again secretes more insulin, and the cycle is perpetuated.

Let us compare diabetes to hypoglycemia. Diabetes includes hypoglycemia in its definition. The unbalanced relationship between blood sugar and insulin is a description of both ailments. It is my belief that diabetes begins first with hypoglycemia, a Greek word that means "low blood sugar." This can be misleading, because it starts with excessive amounts of sugar in the blood. Many people have been suffering from hypoglycemia years before their diabetes is diagnosed. It is so common in the United States that most Americans suffer from it without knowing it.

HYPOGLYCEMIA

Hypoglycemia is extremely common and it afflicts the majority of Americans. Its symptoms include headaches, low energy level, mood swings, alertness, irritability, hunger, tension, and nervousness. Depending upon what food has been ingested, the symptoms can change from hour to hour. Often, hypoglycemia completely controls a patient who is suffering these symptoms, even though he is unaware of it. Many conventional doctors believe there is no such thing as hypoglycemia, categorizing it among those "nonexistent" maladies like PMS or Chronic Fatigue Syndrome. They refuse to admit to it, yet repeatedly they see many patients with the symptoms described above. These physicians do not know how to treat them. The hypoglycemia I refer to and treat with enzymes is not a disease. It is a condition that affects a huge percentage of the population. Most people, if asked, would say they have some of these symptoms. We blindly accept this state of health as a way of life. Remember, low blood sugar is not a diagnosis or a disease—it is a response!

What can we do about hypoglycemia? I advise those who come to my office the importance of health education. We must learn to identify the amount of sugar we use, especially those hidden ones. Most of us do not even know they exist. The next step is to replace the body's depleted supply of carb-splitting enzymes. Along with the enzymes, there are certain herbs that assist with the insulin response. Please do not feel that if you have this condition there is no hope. A change of diet with enzyme supplements can do wonders for you. Hypoglycemia involves allergy or substance intolerance. It is very difficult to determine all the different reactions we have to foods. When we discover what they are, it's even more difficult to eliminate them for the rest of our lives. Therefore, as a preventative, I suggest the use of enzymes to aid digestion and stop toxic reactions.

Symptoms of hypoglycemia can be tolerated for brief periods. However, if the blood sugar level remains very low for a prolonged period, then fatigue and dysfunction develop. These can include confusion, hallucinations, convulsions, and even lapsing into a coma. The nervous system is deprived of glucose necessary for metabolic activity. Another normal response to hypoglycemia is a significant increase of epinephrine, a hormone secreted by the adrenal glands. More serious symptoms develop such as increased pulse rate, tachycardia, elevated blood pressure, sweating, and anxiety. Treatment would depend on the primary cause of hypoglycemia.

If this medical problem that stems from an endocrine or liver disease resulting in the decreased secretion of glucose exists, then special dietary changes are in order. These changes are aimed at avoiding extremes in the blood glucose level by maintaining a constant one at all times. This diet is high in protein and fat, but low in carbohydrates. It calls for frequent, small meals during the day, and one before going to bed. Another cause of hypoglycemia is cell damage to the liver. If someone is fasting, the liver is the primary source of glucose to the bloodstream. This can also result in an ability to convert glycogen into glucose. Glycogen is actually formed by and stored in the liver and, to a lesser extent, in the muscles. Glycogen changes to glucose and is sent to various parts of the body as needed. It's been called the animal starch.

Many people have been told, or assumed, that they have hypoglycemia. Our poor eating habits generate it. Another cause may be an inefficient endocrine system or a tumor. Hypoglycemia is recognized and discussed by most people. The majority of cases, however, are simply glucose intolerance rather than a true hypoglycemia. In either case, there must be a change in the diet. The diet must include protein and careful control over the amount of sugars we eat. Some prescription drugs lower blood sugar levels and interfere with the production of insulin. These drugs create a hypoglycemic effect. Hypoglycemia is touted as one of the disorders of the modern age. Because of that, many people tend to dismiss it. In truth, it is more serious than we think.

One of the first things we do for hypoglycemia in the world of enzyme therapy is to fortify the liver. The best choice for this is protease. I always suggest to my clients who have any form of glucose intolerance to make an effort to identify the foods they crave or eat in the greatest amounts. Then, eat several small, low-sugar meals a day. This way, problem foods that should be avoided can be determined. *Refer to the Body Type section to find your type and the appropriate foods for you.* Above all, good digestion is essential. Protease, in the correct proportion, together with amylase must be used in some supplements.

I see clients in person at my office. In addition, I receive calls from people all over the country who ask about biochemical typing and enzyme therapy. I have developed a questionnaire for all of those who seek my help. I utilize this as a tool to assist me in evaluating individual nutritional needs. One of the disorders listed is hypoglycemia. Most people mark it as a symptom they have experienced. I chose "hypoglycemia" over "glucose intolerance" because most people still do not know what that means. However, if you ask an average American what hypoglycemia is, he or she will answer that it is the fatigue felt after eating sugar. This is an example of how trendy hypoglycemia has become in the last few decades.

CASE HISTORY

This brings to mind a child who came to my office one day. His mother was very concerned about his lethargy; he had become a couch potato. He had no interest in sports or school. All he did was watch TV. However, even that did not keep him focused. His parents thought he had a learning disability. They put him through a long series of tests at one of the local children's hospitals only to find he had no learning difficulties. His inability to concentrate, the dizziness, and shaking he was experiencing were still unexplained by the time they came to see me. After reviewing the boy's diet, it did not take long to realize that his system was completely out of balance due to eating far too many simple carbohydrates. He was suffering from all the symptoms of hypoglycemia, or sugar intolerance. He was willing to eat all the foods we suggested, at the proper times, and to take enzymes. I agreed to drop out of the situation if none of it worked. I made an absolute agreement with him; he promised to work with me. I designed a plan for him that started with enzymes first thing in the morning, between meals and with meals. I explained everything to him, so he understood how the enzymes fortified his system. He and his family saw a real difference within three days. This child told me that he actually felt better within 24 hours. He had a complete reversal, and now he is very involved in schoolwork and neighborhood activities.

Once we got things under control, I could show his parents why all the vitamins and minerals they gave their son, and the methods they used to stop him from eating sugar, were ineffective. He suffered an inability to properly digest his food and utilize it as fuel for his body. No amount of vitamins or changes in his habits would work!

Many parents ask me why they should have to keep sweets from themselves and the rest of the family just because their children cannot control how much sugar they eat. Recently a mother complained to me that her child was sneaking sweets into his room. She could not understand why she and her husband were having behavior problems with him. When she asked the child what they could do to help him, he answered, "Just don't buy those things, Mom." Her comment to him was, "Why should the rest of the family suffer just because you have a problem with sweets?" I pointed out to her that a child learns from parents and other adults. In order for a child to know how to control his sugar intake, the parents must first show that they can control theirs. It is inconsiderate to have something in the house that constantly reminds the child of his forbidden foods. By watching the rest of the family indulging in them, the child becomes confused. He cannot help thinking, "If it's okay for them, why can't I have it, too?" or "Why am I being punished?" That child was very intuitive and absolutely correct with his response. It was obvious to both his mother and me that she too had a problem with sugar. She was not willing to give up her own sugar cravings. Otherwise, she would have happily honored her son's request.

We can readily see other people's destructive behaviors without seeing our own. If you feel fatigued, dizzy, lacking in stamina; if you walk into a room only to forget why you went there; if you are speaking to someone and in mid-sentence, you forget what you were saying; it is time for you to look at your sugar intake. I could relate many stories to you, but they are all very similar to those I have told. We do not like to give up that sugar. We think we feel better when we have it. We do not like to deny ourselves, yet America is asleep because we are eating so much sugar. It is all too easy to justify our behavior by saying we have hypoglycemia, and therefore cannot control our sugar cravings. The truth is, we do not know how to push away those desserts offered to us! In my own experience, by taking plant enzymes for complete carbohydrate digestion, the cravings have lessened because I am allowing my system to heal. Try a program of supplemental digestive enzymes that contain the carbohydrate-splitting enzymes and see what happens.

DETOXIFY AND FORTIFY: PURIFYING YOUR BLOOD... LOWERING YOUR CHOLESTEROL

Detoxify means to counteract or destroy toxins or to remove their effects from the system. In the past, these two processes were employed in a linear fashion. First, by some detoxification process like fasting, we would flush toxins into the blood stream. This caused flu-like symptoms—fever, fatigue, and overall aching. Then we would fortify the body with certain nutrients to restore the balance. Now with enzymes, we can detoxify and fortify at the same time without the side effects. Chapter Three explained exactly how enzymes can be used to cleanse the body and boost good health simultaneously. Enzyme-cleansing eliminates the discomforts associated with detoxification while increasing a sense of well-being and higher energy levels. Enzymes are beautiful and non-invasive ways to cleanse and nourish.

By now you know how strong digestion, combined with a tough immune system, contributes to a healthy, vital blood supply. I have covered many of the reasons why these systems are often below par, allowing the blood to become weak and polluted. It is important to know that germs and viruses only thrive on decaying matter (toxins). They do not attack clean, toxin-free blood, tissues, or organs. Therefore, if we reduce the number of contaminants in our blood, we automatically reduce the number of germs and viruses. There are two ways we can accomplish this. We can depend on the body's ability to cure it, and we can offer a little assistance to get the job done.

Our bodies are true marvels of creation. Hundreds of interconnected organs and systems are programmed to respond to an endless variety of circumstances—good and bad. For example, four major command centers are constantly working to remove toxins from our blood. You will discover that our bowels, kidneys, lungs, and skin (yes, skin!) consider themselves protectors of our blood, among other things. They work tirelessly at keeping the blood free of unwanted debris, each in their own unique way. Unfortunately, when our bodies are short on enzymes, these wonder-workers are not always effective because of the stress we impose on our systems. As we get older, our bodies simply cannot effectively detoxify our blood and lymphatic system without help. The lymphatic system filters out waste products. For example, white blood cells attack bacteria. As part of the process, they die along with the bacteria. The lymphatic system ushers both these waste products to the lymph glands where the fragments break down and assimilate harmlessly into the body. For decades, millions of concerned consumers have tried a variety of self-administered ways to detoxify. They experimented with everything—macrobiotic and other vegetarian diets, fasting, and herbal regimens. Most of these approaches work to some degree, especially the herbal treatments. However, my studies have convinced me that enzyme supplements are the missing ingredient. When taken consistently, they purify the blood by breaking down its undigested proteins, cellular debris, and other toxins. With the blood healthy once again, the body gradually rebuilds itself and replenishes its storehouse of enzymes. The ultimate result: A balanced body capable of functioning at peak efficiency.

I find it interesting that when dealing with people I know, either friends or family, it is very difficult to advise them about their nutritional well-being. It is amusing to learn that you simply cannot tell people whom you know, what to do! I am addressing this because I have suggested the use of enzymes and dietary changes to my own family and close friends. In keeping with our human nature, they all wait until they have manifested a condition or illness before they make any changes. When they finally do take action, it is invariably the result of what they have learned from someone else's book or work. My word to the wise is, if you have found the answers to a loved one's health problems in this book, they may not be ready to listen to your pointing it out to them. Be comfortable with what you have learned—the best example for your friends or family is to see you working diligently at staying healthy. When family and friends do rid their diets of sugar, the results that manifest are so encouraging. Because our nation has such a sweet tooth, we have become so enzyme-deficient that we cannot recognize the battle raging within our bodies. The symptoms are so numerous now that there is a great deal of crossover into other maladies besides sugar addiction. Fatigue, aches, pains, depression, and inflammation describe a multitude of disorders.

One of my relatives recently read a book about Crohn's disease. He is having a problem with his colon and the book detailed the number of malnutrition dilemmas we are facing because our metabolic enzyme output is so badly hindered. The digestive system is so compromised that this colon disorder has now manifested as Crohn's disease. My loved one eliminated almost all the simple carbohydrates, desserts, breads, and some of the pasta from his diet. It worked for him and now he feels so much better. It does not matter whether he heard it from another source or me, the important thing is he understands what he had been doing to himself, and he has taken steps to change his lifestyle. I reiterate, I cannot emphasize too strongly the importance of eliminating sugar or foods that turn into glucose from your diet. Get rid of those sweets, those white breads, and tortillas, and start giving enzymes to your body. I am speaking to myself just as much as to anyone else.

Eating foods that create residue in the small intestine inhibits your metabolic enzymes. This waste matter keeps the villi from absorbing nutrients. The system can no longer depend on the metabolic enzymes, which have been rendered useless. They are unable to respond if called upon, because of the toxic conditions we have created by eating the wrong foods day after day, year after year. The protocol for a very toxic colon that can involve explosive diarrhea calls for the return of a good pH balance. It is almost impossible to achieve if you are nutrient-deficient. If your small and large intestines have bacteria or fungal-form takeover, the best recourse is to use *L. Plantarum*, a natural bacterium. I then call in my protease—the big detoxifier. Protease is a scavenger for improper proteins. Its miraculous properties cannot be praised enough.

Occasionally, you may find someone whose gastrointestinal system is so irritated that taking high doses of protease may cause a slight uncomfortable sensation. (If that is the case, simply take your protease with a meal or small amount of food instead of on an empty stomach.) Most of the time, I find people not drinking enough water when swallowing the capsules. All protease, whether it is metabolic your body makes or supplemental you take orally, require water to work. The other thought is to calm down and repair the system. The bacterium, L. Plantarum, will not create the discomfort. It will restore the natural pH with the "good" bacteria. When this takes place, it works like a natural antibiotic because the body is able to make its own reserves. The next best enzymes for this are high amounts of lipase along with the carbohydrate-splitting enzymes. A good enzyme formulation is what I would use until everything is back to normal.

To be toxic means we have self-poisoned our bodies either with undigested food or through autointoxication. This means we have poisoned our system through toxins locked in the blood stream from something we have not digested properly. Toxins are trapped in our colon where they leak into the blood, and then we have to deal with the adverse effects. There are 36 poisons released into the blood from undigested foods. These poisons, or toxins, are substances that have been ingested, inhaled, absorbed, or have developed within the body. Even in relatively small amounts, they can cause structural damage or functional disturbances.

CHOLESTEROL... IS IT REALLY THE BAD GUY?

We have known for decades that over time, a high-fat diet will raise the cholesterol level in the blood and increase risk of a heart attack. We have also known that unless you are a smoker or have a genetic defect, you have the ability to reduce your cholesterol level. More recently, we have learned that when you reduce your cholesterol level, you also reduce the amount of high-density lipoprotein in the blood. This is not ideal, because HDL plays a very important role. It drives excess cholesterol from the bloodstream into the liver, which removes it from the body. Fortunately, regular exercise offsets the loss of HDL good fats caused by low-fat diets. We often overlook the fact that the body manufactures its own fats. Although we need a certain amount of fat to maintain good health, it is all too easy to accumulate harmful levels. Knowing our individual body type and the foods we should eat is very helpful in preventing our system from overproducing our supply of bad fats.

In spite of our best intentions, however, a majority of us have too many undigested fats floating in our blood. It is very rare for me to find fat-free blood when I view samples under the microscope. The presence of excess fats in the blood is the result of too much fat intake or fat production, too little exercise, or a deficiency of the digestive enzyme lipase, which breaks down fats. Nearly everyone whose blood samples I have evaluated is lipase-deficient. Taking lipase enzyme supplements with every meal easily remedies this.

As a clinical nutritionist, I have no doubt in my mind that good nutrition is the best method of prevention. The general public, because it is uneducated when it comes to good nutrition, views this way of life as too simplistic. For example, the press constantly feeds us information from doctors and government health reports. Because we all pay such close attention to the media, most of us believe that cholesterol causes heart disease, and that we will prevent heart disease by avoiding cholesterol. I believe that no true scientist genuinely believes it. Even though what we hear is just opinion, we have been left with the idea that cholesterol is bad for us.

IS CHOLESTEROL BAD, OR IS IT NECESSARY?

Our bodies manufacture 1,500 milligrams of cholesterol per day. If we do not eat foods containing it, our livers make it for us. This tells me that cholesterol is important. To preserve that all-important state of homeostasis, I believe cholesterol must be in balance with blood sugar, blood pressure, sodium, potassium, and electrolytes. Levels of cholesterol can vary depending on what is driving it. If your good cholesterol (HDL) is driving it due to exercise and everything else is in range, then that is a good cholesterol reading. If triglycerides (LDL) are driving the number, that is not a good reading. Recently warnings have been going out that the low cholesterols have just as many problems as high and can be an indicator of disease. The only problem with this is so many are on cholesterol lowering drugs that falsify or skew the results.

What do triglycerides look like? They are waxy, fat-like substances. When we look at live blood just after someone has eaten or while they are digesting, we expect to see a certain amount of cholesterol floating around in the plasma. If it is not there, we know a big imbalance exists, one that needs correcting as soon as possible. Cholesterol is essential to good health because it is a major building block. It is a component for all the body's hormones, particularly the sex hormones. It plays a major role in the endocrine system and helps form the protective myelin sheath around nerve endings. It also helps in the provision of bile salts for digestion.

I have read cholesterol research and wasn't surprised to find a study done in America with people having blood-cholesterol levels anywhere from 200 to 225 milligrams lived longer than those with levels of 150 to 200 milligrams. That makes a statement that differs greatly from what the media tells us. I have consulted some of my medical doctor colleagues who are more comfortable when their patients' readings are higher than 150 to 200. We know that a certain amount of cholesterol is very important for the maintenance of good health. However, that amount will vary depending on biochemical type. It is intriguing to me that no-fat and low-fat foods are all high in sugars, and many times synthetic sugars, which is a devastating combination. After all, the balance of the cholesterol readings is what is important. Your total cholesterol might be high because your good fats HDL are higher than the range given. This also determines your risk. The higher the HDL levels to the LDL, the lesser the risk.

This is a primary example of trading one problem for another. Many physicians tell me they like how our clinic uses cholesterol readings as indicators of possible nutrition problems. They are not surprised if cholesterol levels are high in patients with heart disease. Rather, they are concerned that this indicates the causes for both high cholesterol and heart disease are the same. It is sugar consumption more so than fatty foods, which drive up cholesterol levels, because sugar causes the liver to make large amounts of triglycerides. A lethal combination is a donut (fried starch!)

In my office, as in those of countless health professionals using enzyme therapy, high or low cholesterol is not a problem. I say that with complete confidence. Whether clients suffer from high cholesterol because of an inherited condition or create high cholesterol through improper diet, they are given a formulation high in lipase, along with other supportive enzymes, and Brindall Berry combined with other herbs. Their high cholesterol level can drop within a 21-day period. Laboratory tests, university findings, and our research support this fact. Immune-deficient clients with low cholesterol are also brought into the normal, healthy range with enzyme supplements. For some it happens even more quickly when they make positive dietary changes.

It is important to discuss the research on high-cholesterol foods. The information available to most of us tells us that we should not eat eggs or animal fats because of their high cholesterol content. Even though it has been proven that eggs do not present a cholesterol problem, we are still told not to eat them. It is worthwhile to investigate whom the sponsors are of the tests that are run and how the information is delivered to an unsuspecting public. I feel it is not in our best interests to stop eating eggs, because they are very high in necessary amino acids. We hear that cholesterol will escape into the blood, lining the blood vessels with the harmful plaque that creates heart disease. The real truth is that the cholesterol (yoke) when eaten with the white (amino acids) causes greater balance and use of the protein. Nature does not make mistakes—just man.

EAT THE WHOLE EGG

Many doctors will now tell you that cholesterol does not create plaque as much as it is the presence of "free radicals" (next paragraph). I personally advise Body Type One to start the morning with eggs. It amuses me how many people question the cholesterol content in eggs. I show my clients the documented research so they can be comfortable with knowing that the egg is safe to eat. I consider the egg white to be one of the ideal protein sources. Cholesterol is only present in the egg yolk. However, it is the synergy between the egg white and the yolk that makes an egg such a superior protein source. They are the healthy lipoprotein that balances the good cholesterol. Clinically, eggs are highly nutritious, because they contain important amino acids. Science uses the egg as a standard measure for all protein when eating the whole egg. If a health professional advises that eggs are bad for you, as an allergy to eggs, then of course they could be harmful for you. This could be a warning that perhaps your body is not making the correct amount of protease and lipase. When I recommend certain foods to a client, I always make sure the foods are eaten with the right amount of enzyme supplements to assure proper digestion. For me, any concern with cholesterol would begin with looking at lipase activity. Next, I would consider the body's ability to handle lipids, and what should be done to balance the body type with foods and enzymes.

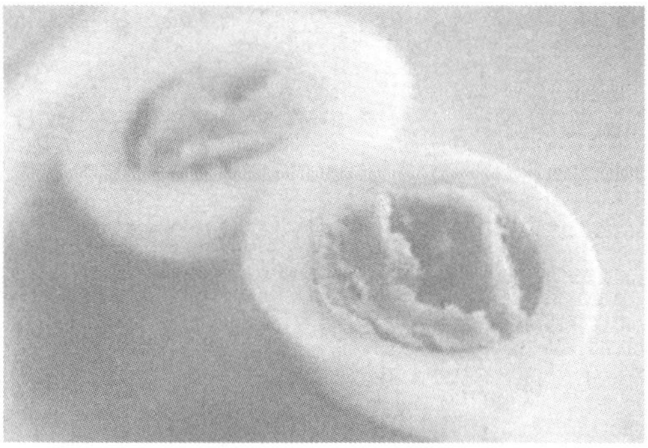

WHAT PART DOES CHOLESTEROL PLAY IN THE CREATION OF PLAQUE?

Does it arrive early or late in the procedure? Was it formed because of eating a high-cholesterol food, or was it brought on because junk food seems to encourage the production of free radicals? Dr. Elmer Cranton, President of the American Holistic Medicine Association and author of "Bypassing Bypass," was the first to propose a theory that has influenced the thinking of many health professionals. He suggests that perhaps the role of cholesterol is to help protect the body from free-radical oxidation. Cholesterol is one of the body's natural antioxidants. This means the body manufactures it to guard against the oxidizing damage by free radicals. While sheltering the afflicted area, cholesterol is converted to its oxidized form, which is harmful to the blood cells. The HDLs counteract this effect. LDLs are associated more closely with heart disease than with total cholesterol.

In the nutrition field, many have concluded that cholesterol is not the enemy. High-serum cholesterol (LDL) results from the imbalance in the body. Enzyme antioxidants, along with vitamins found naturally in herbs, are the answer to the body's need for nutrients with which to rebuild itself. The media bombards us with information about popular antioxidants on today's market. Pine bark or grape seed, which I prefer, are two of them. Rose hips are better than synthetic vitamin C. Alfalfa is another product that works well in the restorative process. Siberian ginseng is a nutrient as well as an antioxidant. I use Ginkgo biloba leaf and extract regularly. Remember, the strongest scavenger is protease. Another enzyme is lipase, which delivers other antioxidants into the bloodstream. With a correct formulation of all these enzymes, herbs, and nutrients, the invaders do not stand a chance!

OBESITY IS A BIG PROBLEM IN AMERICA (PUN INTENDED)

In 2012 over 34.2 percent of Americans were overweight and another 33.7 percent were obese. Do you realize this comes to 67.9 percent of Americans being FAT! We spend over $147,000 per year on exercise and diet pills, all because we are trying to get rid of the fat cells in our bodies. After we spend all that money, most of our efforts fail, and lost pounds are usually found once again. Visit any newsstand or magazine section of a supermarket and you will notice that almost every book or magazine features an article on weight loss, a new way to build the body, or a breakthrough diet. All of these books and articles say much of the same thing. There is disagreement regarding low fat, more protein, no protein, or all vegetables. It seems no one takes the time to explain to the public that the greatest imbalance is enzyme imbalance. One form of help for weight loss touted is diet pills, either prescription or over-the-counter. Usually these pills contain an appetite suppressant that helps you cut back on your food until you can get control of it. Others are made up of medications that block insulin production and deter us from addressing another function of our metabolism.

However, when we stop taking the pills, the weight always comes back. Most of these medications have side effects, so they can be taken for only short periods of time. Consider the terrible side effects of Fen-Phen, thermal medicine, or ephedrine supplements. For some people, a lifelong weight problem means a continuous cycle of gain and loss that puts an incredible amount of stress on our bodies as well as our emotions. Whatever the situation, shedding excess pounds is indeed a difficult task. What is more, the road to a slender body is paved with nutritional dangers. Most diets fall short when it comes to providing adequate nutrition. The HCL diet is now under the gun for the amount of calories being under what is considered healthy. Some diets suggest certain foods or food groups, while others say to eliminate this food and try that one. The most critical point to remember is that each cell in your body requires 45 different nutrients to remain healthy! An article published in the New England Journal of Medicine stated that research has proved both men and women who diet frequently suffer from heart disease more often than others.

To make matters worse, habitual dieting is a setup for weight gain. While you eat less to lose unwanted fat, your body thinks it is starving. It has a natural survival mechanism that allows it to cling to calories or fat, making weight loss even more difficult. If a diet recommends less than 1,200 calories a day, it will not provide adequate nutrients. I know you have heard all this before. What you may not know is that people are overweight because they cannot properly digest food efficiently or receive delivery of the nutrients to their cells. Therefore, the body cries out for more and more food. To answer that call, we eat more without assimilating anything of value and gain even more weight. One can be overweight or obese and be nutrient deficient.

Enzyme supplements added to a meal will help the foods through the digestive process, finally delivering the nutrients. Enzymes taken between meals will assist with cleanup of undigested food particles. Enzymes are critical for the treatment of obesity. Overweight people unable to control food cravings continue to assault their bodies and immune systems with high-calorie foods that are devoid of nutritional value. Plant-based enzymes solve these problems and keep us from doing any further harm to our health.

On June 20, 2013, the American Medical Association (AMA) declared obesity a disease, effectively making it a medical condition requiring treatment!

Here is a good question that we should be asking—who is going to treat these now nearly 80 million obese American adults and 15 million obese American children now in need of medical treatment? According to the AMA, it should be physicians. Which is an odd choice since obesity is intimately linked with—if not directly related to—eating and exercise behavior. And throughout their training, most medical students receive less than two weeks' curriculum in nutrition prescription and no direct coursework in exercise prescription. Of course, obesity isn't just about eating properly and exercising. In many cases, obese individuals have lifestyle-related metabolic or hormonal disturbances that also need to be addressed.

Of course, obesity isn't just about eating properly and exercising. In many cases, obese individuals have lifestyle-related metabolic or hormonal disturbances that cause them not to properly digest their food, utilize the nutrients, and metabolically turn it into energy—creating more storage of fat in the cells. According to Dr. Spencer Nadolsky, a practicing physician in Virginia who works with many overweight and obese clients, "The average physician is taught next to nothing about obesity treatment in medical school and residency." Beyond the obvious lack of training preventing most physicians from being able to effectively treat obesity, there's another issue at stake: **physicians just aren't afforded enough time with their patients.** Recent research suggests that the average amount of time American physicians spend with their patients is eight minutes; barely enough time for a presentation of symptoms and a subsequent referral or prescription. "When a patient is overweight or obese," says Dr. Nadolsky, "every doctor's knee jerk response is to mention 'diet and exercise.'" Sure, we've all heard it before. But let's be honest, **"eat right and exercise" is nothing more**

than a cliché. Like a mother wagging her finger and telling children to eat their vegetables, it has no teeth.

Which brings us back to the original question: If physicians have:

- Essentially no training in nutrition and exercise prescription for obesity,
- Minimal training in the relationship between metabolic health and obesity,
- Very little time to actually discuss lifestyle intervention in obesity, then
- Who's going to treat obesity?

The answer may be in the obese person's own hands. We have to learn what causes this disease and stop doing it. It is called overeating of improper foods for our own individual health. I know it is easier said than done, but it is up to the individual to do it just like any other disease on this planet.

Every person needs to pay attention to the food he or she puts in his or her body, properly digest this food, rid the body of toxins, and maintain balance in our 100 trillion cells for energy, metabolism, and health. We may lack the specific enzymes to properly breakdown our foods, thereby challenging our immune system, which is located in our digestive tract; and compromise our liver, lungs, kidneys, and skin by the inability to rid ourselves of the buildup of toxins.

PERFECT STORM OF INFLAMMATION PROMOTES WEIGHT GAIN AND DIABETES

A wide array of health problems, including but not limited to obesity, insulin resistance, type II diabetes, periodontal disease, stroke, and heart disease, all have inflammation as a part of the disease.

The majority of inflammatory diseases start in your gut. Chronic inflammation in your gut can disrupt the normal functioning of many bodily systems. There also appears to be a connection between certain types of bacteria and body fat that produces a heightened inflammatory response and drives the inflammatory process.

Your Digestive System may be making you fat! It's hard to believe—but very true. I want to explain that poorly digested food, along with improper bacteria in your digestive tract, upset your gut's immune system and how they just might be behind those extra pounds.

I have observed this phenomenon in hundreds of patients. Recently, remarkable new research has confirmed this perfect storm of inflammation. I have mentioned effective treatments for the gut, the immune system, detoxification system, hormones, and more and explained how the systems are connected. For example, I've seen patients who lose significant amounts of weight, just by cutting food allergens from their diet. And I have also seen people lose 20 to 30 pounds simply by balancing the bacterial ecosystem in their intestinal system.

One patient, a 39-year-old woman, had chronic inflammation, fluid retention, acne, fatigue, joint pain, as well as irritable bowel syndrome with bloating and gas. She had tried every known diet but was unable to lose weight.

She could not lose weight because she was inflamed. The imbalances in her gut and the food sensitivities resulted in this "perfect storm of inflammation." But when we had her eliminate the foods to which she was allergic or sensitive and gave her supplemental digestive enzymes to properly break down her food, along with healthy probiotics to heal her gut, she lost 35 pounds in a few months—and all her other symptoms went away!

A big debate in nutrition is which comes first: inflammation or obesity. I have always believed that we become inflamed first and gain weight second—which makes us even more inflamed, perpetuating the cycle.

Now incredible new research bears this out. Previous research has shown that obese people have different intestinal bacteria than slim people. Lean people tend to have higher amounts of various healthy or beneficial bacteria compared to those who carry a lot of excess weight and who tend to have greater colonization of pathogenic bacteria.

For instance, the human adenovirus-36—a cause of respiratory infections and pinkeye—might play a role in promoting obesity by transforming adult stem cells into fat cells that are capable of storing additional fat.

Researchers have also discovered that certain gut bacteria, including Staphylococcus aureus (staph) and E. coli, trigger fat cells to produce inflammatory cytokines. Researchers have proposed that this interaction can provoke the development of diabetes, which is a well-known "side effect" of obesity. Staph bacteria in particular appear to play an important role in diabetes, and according to the featured article, there are two primary reasons for this: Obese people have a tendency to become heavily colonized with staph bacteria.

Staph bacteria are the most common bacteria found in diabetic foot ulcers.

Previous studies have come to similar conclusions. For example, one study found that babies with high numbers of Bifidobacterium (beneficial bacteria) and low numbers of Staphylococcus aureus, appeared to be protected from excess weight gain. This may also be one reason why breast-fed babies have a lower risk of obesity, as Bifidobacterium flourish in the guts of breast-fed babies.

FOR OPTIMAL HEALTH, ADDRESS AND AVOID CHRONIC INFLAMMATION

Remember, the microorganisms living in your digestive tract form a very important "inner ecosystem" that influences countless aspects of health. More specifically, the type and quantity of organisms in your gut interact with your body in ways that can either prevent or encourage the development of chronic inflammation, which is at the heart of many diseases, including heart disease and diabetes. The composition of your microflora may even dictate the ease with which you're able to shed unwanted pounds.

Since virtually all of us are exposed to factors that destroy beneficial bacteria in your gut, such as antibiotics (whether you take them for an illness or get them from contaminated animal products), chlorinated water, antibacterial soap, agricultural chemicals, and pollution, ensuring your gut bacteria remain balanced, should be considered an ongoing process.

When you eat a bad diet, bad bacteria flourish. Your whole gut ecosystem is upset and the outside world "leaks" in across a damaged gut lining.

TESTIMONIALS

"Rome's Biggest Loser"

Dr. DicQie Fuller-Looney provides the most effective supplements for digestive health in the world. We have had tremendous success helping people restore normal digestive function with the constant usage of her Probiotic, Digest, and Protease. In conjunction with a healthy diet and supplemental enzymes, amazing things can happen. We have also had amazing success reducing joint and muscle inflammation with her combination of systemic Protease for inflammation and another product for repair of muscle, tissues, and bone.

I currently use these products with the world-class-sprinters that I coach. There is absolutely no substitution for these products!

We had our first meeting with the Rome's Biggest Loser contestants. I took a poll regarding digestive health. Out of 20 contestants:

- *11 had their gallbladders removed*

- *6 complained of constipation (1 had a complete blockage and had to drop out for medical reasons*
- *16 said they suffered from frequent gas, bloating, and indigestion*

After two weeks almost every person was asymptomatic. There were very few complaints of indigestion, frequent bloating, and gas. The combination of Protease, Digest, and Probiotic ensured that each contestant would be able to digest, assimilate, and use the nutrients they were consuming. Without these enzyme products, it would have been impossible for the contestants to lose such a large amount of weight in just six weeks.

One participant made the following comment: "I was lucky enough to be chosen as one of the participants in the program. Whether or not I am the ultimate winner of the competition, I have already won by losing over 15 pounds in six weeks. I have used many supplements over the years, but not often for weight loss. Your efforts to ensure digestion health are very much appreciated! I was eating a lot of food, and I am sure that your products helped me digest it efficiently. I will be sure to recommend your products to anyone seeking good digestive health."

"Dr. Fuller, I personally want to thank you *for your work and how attentive you were to me while suffering with my gallbladder. As you know, I spent years looking for an answer to my nausea and diarrhea. Just at the time I was ready to give up and have my gallbladder removed (even had a surgery date) I heard of you. It was so refreshing to be educated on why my problem existed and suggestions on what to do. I wanted to believe your supplements would make a difference, but I had tried so many things, even other enzyme products. I followed your protocol and in 24 hours felt a difference that I was afraid to even talk about. Here I am all these years later having cancelled my surgery and doing absolutely fine. The only thing I ask of you is to make sure I can always get your products." - W Brink - Denver, CO*

"Our son is 9 years old *and was diagnosed with Autism several years ago. We first began working on his diet and saw improvements. Then we started giving him digestive enzymes and probiotics, and he got even better. Now we have added the Carbo-G and it is the perfect combination. And we will not stop them. Our son's concentration and* *awareness is better. He takes direction without a struggle and follows through on tasks. He is less 'moody' and is happier. There is a definite difference for the better!" - L Esquivel, MD - San Antonio, TX*

***"I was at a business luncheon** that included a buffet. They had regular bread and gluten-free bread available, so I chose the gluten-free bread since I am very gluten sensitive. I hadn't eaten a sandwich in over a year, so I was really excited about my lunch. I was almost completely finished eating when I realized the bread had been mixed up and I had actually eaten the regular bread. I had already taken my usual dosage of enzymes with my meal but quickly took 3 more Carbo-G. Later that night and the next day, I experienced very little if any of my usual gluten issues. I slept well and had no brain fog, headaches, or stomach issues the next day. It was amazing!" - D Aubrey, CCN, CNC*

***"My granddaughter** loved the Carbo-G. She isn't very compliant and I am trying to work with her on taking it more often. I have also been giving it to people who travel and might not know for sure they are eating gluten free. I am very excited about the product and looking forward to getting more patients on it." - C Brinkley, RN - Henderson, NC*

***"I have started with** six patients on Carbo-G now as part of their protocol. I was planning on them taking it for six weeks before I retest their serum values. The subjective feedback so far is positive. All of them are experiencing less bloating than before. Three of the six are endurance athletes and are experiencing less GI stress from their glycogen replacements supplements on their long runs when they use Carbo-G before their training sessions. After six weeks on Carbo-G, there is a 7 percent average drop in both AGA and IGG antibody tests and a 16.3 average drop in CRP. I have about three more weeks before I start pulling more labs and I will know more then." - C Banks, DC - Texas*

NOTES

- Before putting a product on the market we ask doctors to perform tests on their patients who volunteer. The above testimony reflects the testing period using the volunteer's blood
- **AGA** stands for anti gliadin antibodies, which are antibodies produced by the body in response to contact with gliadin, a part of the gluten molecule.
- **IgG** stands for immunoglobulin G, which are generalized antibody molecules.
- **C-reactive protein (CRP)** is a protein found in the blood, the levels of which rise in response to inflammation.

RENEWAL PROGRAM (BEGINNER)

It takes a committed effort to renew the body itself.

What it requires:

- Knowledge of foods that will promote energy and renewal of our system
- Knowledge of foods that will promote healthy tissue, bone, and muscle building
- A plan for what to eat and how often
- Exercise to refurbish the body and improve how we feel
- Adequate pure water intake to bathe our cells and eliminate waste
- Proper length of the program to allow for rebuilding—anywhere from three to six weeks before moving into the Advanced Program.

Those that need the renewal program:

Anyone who is or has been out of balance (for an ongoing period of time), which has created imbalance within his or her body system itself such as:

- Cancer patients
- People diagnosed with conditions (system or organ dysfunction)
- Obesity / overeating
- Depression / anxiety
- Fatigue / confusion

"Transformational Renewal" how to do it:

- Renew and feel good while doing it
- Know what takes place when you begin the renewal of all systems
- Proper eating and exercise will promote energy throughout all systems of the body during each step of the Renewal Program
- A simple one-page system for every day

MOODS / EMOTION AND EXERCISE

A brisk 10-minute walk will increase energy and improve mood for up to two hours with decreased tension as a secondary effect.

Exercise scientists from two universities studied 93 well-educated women for 11 weeks and noted that when they exercised (leisurely, brisk walk or yoga) for 20 minutes they would self-rate themselves as revitalized (expressed as feelings of energized, refreshed, and revitalized).

Secondary, they felt happy feelings and joyfulness plus increased positive mood changes.

Third, they had a feeling of tranquility, calmness, peacefulness, and relaxation.

However, when exercise scientist Nicholaas Pronk at Texas A&M University monitored 23 same-type women, working them harder at a moderate or demanding rate of exercise for 22 minutes, they noted that mood changes grew worse (as in tension, anxiety, and exhaustion). After an hour the anxiety began to decrease.

For recovery, any moderate to difficult exercise is not to be attempted, as this will create catabolism (breakdown) rather than renewal.

When you burn glucose too fast through strenuous exercise, you begin catabolism. Long, slow exercise burns the fat and does not break down the muscle.

This program encourages body renewal.

IT IS IMPORTANT NOT TO LOSE MUSCLE MASS NEEDED TO RENEW THE BODY

Keep in mind when you want to build (anaerobic) you cannot do so from a catabolic state (tearing down). Breaking down is not a building state for your body.

Negative moods will influence your ability to heal and rebuild (renew) your body.

Negative emotions influence eating wrong foods for recovery and show up as an absence of energy at the cell.

I quote Dr. Dick Couey: "You might want to include the science of the integral protein membranes which are found in our cells. They open when you have a positive attitude, and close down when you have a negative attitude. They open the widest when you have a good belly laugh. Maybe, laughter is the best medicine. Also, they close down when you are angry or fearful. They can also open when you pray."

PROPER FOOD FOR RENEWAL

Carbohydrates break down to glucose, which fuels our muscles and brain. Glucose assisted by insulin is escorted into cells by enzymes. Once inside the cell, glucose is quickly metabolized to energy. Or, if you eat more than is needed, glucose can be converted to either liver or muscle glycogen, which we use during exercise for energy. However, if our metabolism has been negatively compromised, it will be stored as fat.

CARBOHYDRATES ARE IN THE FOLLOWING CATEGORIES:

Simple Carbohydrates/Starches are those that are quickly converted to glucose and they include sugars, breads, cereals, desserts, jam/jelly, and fruit juice (processed foods). Excess consumption of these foods causes an over-stimulated release of insulin, which activates fat cell enzymes to bring the glucose in for storage or make additional fat cells as needed. Remember, if it is packaged, it has additives and is usually a simple carbohydrate/starch.

Complex Carbohydrates are those that are slowly converted to glucose. They include high fiber foods, sprouted grain breads such as Ezekiel 4:9 bread, yams, Quinoa, (rice brown, wild & long grain), beans and most fresh vegetables and greens. Consumption of these foods creates less of an insulin spike and when combined with protein, there is a desired slow, steady release of energy.

When carbohydrate and protein foods are in short supply, the body will begin to break down its own muscle for energy, which can become dangerous to our overall health.

WRONG FOODS INFLUENCE POOR MOODS, BUT PROPER FOODS INFLUENCE RECOVERY

Proper foods for renewal are complex carbohydrates (slow-burning glucose). Fats should be eaten in their natural form. No low-in-fat or low-in-sugar products. These are man-made and incomplete. Low-in-fat or low-in-sugar simply means high in "synthetic" sugar. Proteins break down to amino acids and cannot be stored in the body like sugars or fat.

Avoid synthetic sugar completely as it will sabotage your success!

Plant foods are lower in the amino acids (the building blocks of protein) that are required for re-building of tissue and for growth and repair. It is very difficult to obtain enough protein (all the amino acids required by the cell) from plant sources such as soy, legumes, or nuts. They need to be combined with another food to give you the complete amino acids that are demanded by the cell. An example is rice and beans eaten at the same time. Our bodies do not store proteins for use later on.

EATING FOR RENEWAL

PROTEINS IN OUR DIETS

Protein in our diets comes from both animal and vegetable sources. Most animal sources (meat, milk, eggs, fowl, and fish) provide what's called "complete protein", meaning that they contain all of the essential amino acids. Vegetable sources usually are low on or missing certain essential amino acids. For example, rice is low in isoleucine and lysine. Though different vegetable sources are deficient in different amino acids, you should understand that by combining different foods you can get most of the essential amino acids throughout the course of the meal. Some vegetable sources such as nuts, beans, and soybeans are all fairly high in protein. By combining them, you can get pretty good coverage of essential amino acids. I no longer suggest soy because they are almost all genetically modified, and their estrogen abilities are not suitable for men (men's boobies) or women with cancer.

Protein food is the highest metabolic food. For renewal you need at least 3 oz. for a female and 4 oz. for a male per meal.

The most complete proteins (bearing 8 - 9 amino acids) are lean meat, poultry, fish, and/or eggs. One egg equals 1 oz. of protein. These are complete amino acid sources. One scoop of whey protein isolate and/or natural whey should represent 3 - 4 oz. of protein. Organic products are preferred and should include grass-fed beef, organic poultry, and fresh caught or wild fish.

Protein of choice is grass-fed lean animal meat such as poultry (chicken or turkey), fish (wild salmon or tuna), lean beef, and eggs. Choose organic, hormone free, and mercury free when available. You may have whey protein powder for snacks. Pork is not recommended.

NOTE: Plant sources such as tofu is made from soy and should not be eaten by anyone with breast cancer, including men, because of their estrogen containing phytoestrogens. It is now difficult to find good soy foods that do not contain genetically modified organisms (GMOs).

Carbohydrates of choice are Organic complexes (slow-burning glucose) and include yams, beans, rice (brown, wild and long grain), most vegetables (including squash), greens (raw), and raw fruit (no fruit juice). Eat organic every opportunity possible.

Starch is not the best carbohydrate source and should be avoided. If you are gluten sensitive, I suggest a specific gluten formula for this in place of the other digestive products.

Proper fats are important food for our hormones and cells. Do not eat fried foods for renewal.

Foods can be boiled grilled, baked, sautéed, or steamed. Vegetables are wonderful in a raw state as in salads or snacks.

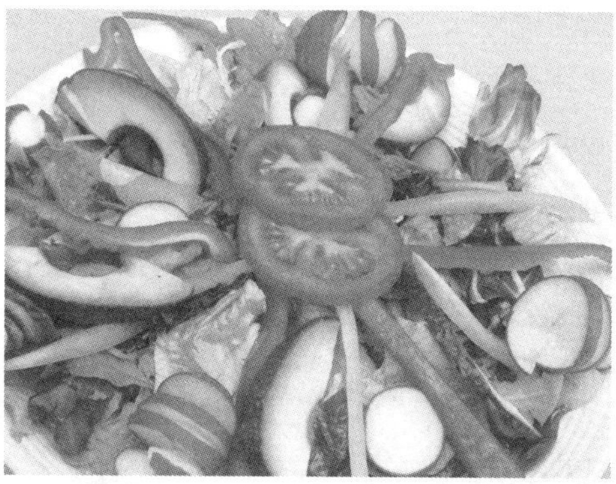

Do not remove the yolk from the egg. It does not make improper fat, and it is the combination of the two substances that add up to the perfect protein food.

The best choices are unsaturated fats that contain omega 3 and a few 6, as these essential fatty acids are found within nuts, seeds, fish oil, avocados, and virgin olive or coconut oil.

Eat protein and carbohydrates at each meal and snack. This is very important to your success.

Remember, when and how often you eat is just as important as what you eat. Eat protein and complex carbohydrates at each meal, or snack every 3 to 3.5 hours during the day.

RENEWAL PROGRAM INCLUDES PROPER EXERCISE AND FOOD FOR REJUVENATION

How it works:

- Exercise at a slow rate for 10 to 20 minutes if you are just beginning, and know that your metabolism increases as glucose is broken down and energy is released as ATP.
- In turn, the mitochondria in our muscles and systems are activated—this takes place at the cellular level in all the systems of our bodies.
- During exercise, heart rate, blood pressure, and respiration increase resulting in more oxygen circulation throughout the entire body.
- Stress hormones such as cortisol and adrenal both influence arousal responses (energy) and are released in the blood stream.
- Neurotransmitters and neuromodulators (norepinephrine and serotonin) are also increased.
- Energy is generated throughout from a pattern of arousal, and feelings of well-being increase that can last for hours.
- Take Protease capsules for repair following your exercise.

Food is for the renewal of cells:

- Eat every 3 to 3.5 hours or six small meals a day
- You must eat at least five times a day for the program to work
- This keeps food in the stomach most of the day (increases metabolism)
- Keeps you from fatigue
- Gives you the building blocks to repair

Metabolism is the sum of all the chemical changes and reactions that happen in your body. Some reactions build up (anabolic) and some tear down (catabolic) and they go on simultaneously every second of your life. The raw material your body uses for metabolism comes from the food you eat and the nutrients the food contains.

The speed that your body does the above tasks is referred to as metabolic rate. Since you have a condition or imbalance, it is likely that yours is very slow or inefficient.

Renewal is about changing your metabolism, improving digestion, and utilizing your food properly.

- When and how often you eat is just as important as what you eat.
- Eat protein and complex carbohydrates at each meal or snack.

Ingest supplemental digestive enzymes with each meal along with pure 8 - 10 oz. of water to activate enzymes.

Sensitive types do best if they ingest a soothing formula of enzymes and a probiotic with meals.

SUGGESTED RENEWAL PLAN

Start the day with breakfast—you must "break" fast.

Breakfast: 3 to 4 egg omelet with vegetables or 2 egg-omelet, and include 2 oz. white organic cheese and one fruit of choice. No fruit juice. Drink 8 - 10 oz. of water along with 1 - 2 capsules of your supplemental plant-based Digestive Formula, plus and an extra Protease capsule.

3 hours later: 4 oz. protein of choice with organic fruit or vegetable, for example a smoothie made with 25 grams of protein powder, ice, and fruit. Drink 8 - 10 oz. of water with Digestive Formula, plus 1 Protease capsule.

3 to 3.5 hours later: Lunch – 4 oz. protein of choice such as chicken salad and greens. Drink 8 - 10 oz. of water with 1 - 2 capsules Digestive Formula, plus 1 Protease capsule.

3 to 3.5 hours later: Snack – 4 oz. of water packed wild tuna or salmon with an apple. Drink 8 - 10 oz. of water with 1 - 2 capsules of Digestive Formula, plus 1 Protease capsule.

3 to 3.5 hours later: Dinner – 4 oz. protein of choice such as lean meat with a yam (sweet potato) and salad. Drink 8 - 10 oz. of water with 1 - 2 capsules of Digestive Formula, plus 1 Protease capsule.

Evening snack (optional): 3 - 4 oz. of protein food with grapefruit* or cup of berries, plus 1 capsule Digestive Formula.

Before bed: 2 - 3 capsules of systemic plant based Protease plus 1 - 2 capsules Probiotic with 8 - 10 oz. of water.

**Make sure your medication does not prohibit grapefruit*

Supplemental enzymes along with metabolic enzymes made by your own body are both hydrolytic and require water to work. You must drink at least 8 oz. of water with enzyme supplements and/or when eating.

RENEWAL PROGRAM (ADVANCED)

In the Beginners' Renewal Program, you learned about food and how to feed the body for renewal. In this program you will learn how the cell renews itself when given the opportunity by not feeding the body system. You might think this an oxymoron, but there are scientific studies to back this up. You may enjoy this program and want to make it an ongoing part of your life.

There is a lot of initial evidence to suggest that temporary periodic fasting can induce long-lasting changes that can be beneficial against aging and diseases.

One of the ways fasting works is by making your body reduce the amount of IGF-1 it produces.

I am speaking of alternate fasts, not a prolonged fast, because there are risks with prolonged fasting.

Chapter 7

Genetically Modified Foods (GMO)

"ALL DISEASE BEGINS IN THE GUT" - HIPPOCRATES

Food for Thought: The Environmental Working Group, a consumer advocate organization, determined that Americans eat, on average, 193 pounds of GMO foods a year. The group justifiably asks: "If you were planning on eating your body weight of anything in a year, wouldn't you want to make sure it was safe to eat?"

Other countries are more concerned about these foods than we are. As a matter of fact, the United States is just about alone in not requiring labeling of GMO foods or the performance of safety tests to see whether these bizarre, chemist-created foods are harmless. As a result, about 90 percent of the corn, soy, and cotton now produced in the United States are GMO crops. When you eat processed foods like corn chips or breakfast cereal, 70 percent of what you take in has been made from GMO products.

WHAT IS ON YOUR PLATE?

These foods consist of genetically modified organisms (GMO)—plants that have been created in laboratories and then planted by farmers. The most frightening part about these foods is that they are unlike any other foods that humans have ever eaten. And they were probably on your dinner plate last night and almost certainly in your snack foods. ***See genetically modified organisms and sugar at the end of this chapter.***

THIS IS NOT A NEW PROBLEM

We started noticing many of our young people coming into the clinic were experiencing abnormal amounts of digestive problems. Twenty years ago I had a radio show in Scottsdale where I started teaching about the genetically modified organisms in our food. One of my subjects was the "new tomatoes" that contained pork genes for stability on the shelf. Our government began using these GMOs in much of our produce and of course since then it has evolved into food that is no longer nutritious. I started the show by recognizing vegetarians that made their decision to be vegetarian based on spiritual beliefs. I asked them if they were aware they may be eating pork genes in their vegetables or insect genes in their fruits.

Now, we are all aware of gluten sensitivities and many diverse gut related dysbiosis (referring to a condition with microbial imbalances on or within the body). Dysbiosis is most prominent in the digestive tract or on the skin, but it can also occur on any exposed surface or mucous membrane such as the vagina, lungs, nose, sinuses, ears, nails, or eyes. It has been associated with different illnesses, like inflammatory bowel disease and chronic fatigue syndrome. Over the years, this has only worsened with the introduction of the genetically altered foods.

I mentioned that we are given everything we need in the first few days of our lives (while yet an embryo). This includes our genetic instructions on how our bodies will handle their proteins. Proteins are extremely important because our bodies makes hormones from them, not only sexual hormones but those needed for our neurotransmitters, signaling systems, repair of cells, tissue, organs, metabolic enzymes, and amino acid chains. The usage and importance of proteins cannot be numbered.

Consider that genetically modified organisms are the DNA (proteins) from animal, insect, fowl, virus, and bacteria, and they are being spliced (interweaved) into our foods. Our bodies do not recognize these proteins from other species and will see them as an allergy. Eighty percent of our immune system resides in our digestive tract (small intestine), and we react to these proteins creating inflammation and allergies. Immune disorders, or the body turning itself on as in autoimmune disorders, are now worsening.

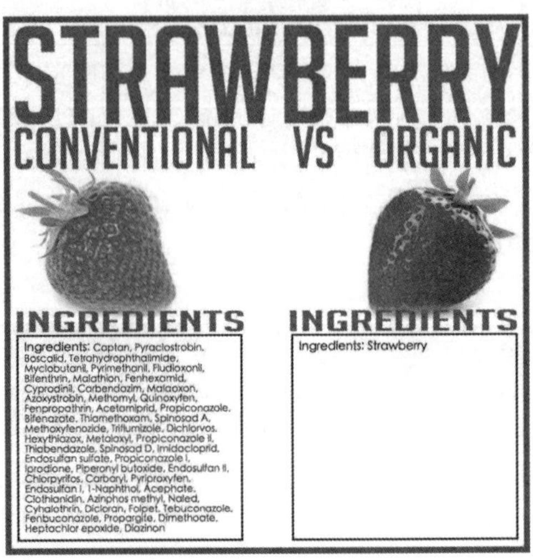
STRAWBERRY
CONVENTIONAL VS ORGANIC
INGREDIENTS
Ingredients: Captan, Pyraclostrobin, Boscalid, Tetrahydrophthalimide, Myclobutanil, Pyrimethanil, Fludioxonil, Bifenthrin, Malathion, Fenhexamid, Cyprodinil, Carbendazim, Malaoxon, Azoxystrobin, Methomyl, Quinoxyfen, Fenpropathrin, Acetamiprid, Propiconazole, Bifenazate, Thiamethoxam, Spinosad A, Methoxyfenozide, Triflumizole, Dichlorvos, Hexythiazox, Metalaxyl, Propiconazole II, Thiabendazole, Spinosad D, Imidacloprid, Endosulfan sulfate, Propiconazole I, Iprodione, Piperonyl butoxide, Endosulfan II, Chlorpyrifos, Carbaryl, Pyriproxyfen, Endosulfan I, 1-Naphthol, Acephate, Clothianidin, Azinphos methyl, Naled, Cyhalothrin, Dicloran, Folpet, Tebuconazole, Fenbuconazole, Propargite, Dimethoate, Heptachlor epoxide, Diazinon
INGREDIENTS
Ingredients: Strawberry

When I first started in practice, autism was recognized as one in a million children, and then it moved to one in 100 thousand until it went to one in 150 children and two years ago it was one in 37 children. It escalated when we started eating the genetically modified foods. We humans do not make digestive enzymes to properly digest these genetically modified foods, and they are creating incredible disorders. This is what the rise of gluten sensitivities are all about since they are a protein mixed with a carbohydrate, which our bodies do not recognize or know what to do with it.

If you want more information you can go online to the USDA site where they are very honest about the genetically modified foods.

The following definitions were taken from Department of Agriculture website:

Genetics: Each person has an estimated 20,000 to 25,000 genes carrying 3 billion bits of information that constitute an instruction book for the body. When some of those bits become scrambled or otherwise distorted, diseases may result. Research has focused on the variations among people that can be used to create new treatments.

Agricultural Biotechnology: A range of tools, including traditional breeding techniques, that alter living organisms, or parts of organisms, to make or modify products; improve plants or animals; or develop microorganisms for specific agricultural uses. Modern biotechnology today includes the tools of genetic engineering.

Genetic engineering: Scientists borrow a gene found naturally in one organism—called the donor—and supply it to a second organism called the recipient. Scientists usually perform the exchange in a manner that ensures that the recipient organism will naturally pass the new gene along to its offspring.

Manipulation of an organism's genes by introducing, eliminating, or rearranging specific genes using the methods of modern molecular biology, particularly those techniques referred to as recombinant DNA techniques.

Allergen: A substance, usually a protein, which can cause an allergy or allergic reaction in the body.

Allergy: A reaction by the body's immune system after exposure to a particular substance, often a protein.

I do hope you go to the site and see for yourself. There are many good books written about GMOs and some eye-opening DVDs. Go online or on Amazon and look at the ones that you would be most interested in reading.

My degrees in nutrition and health science no longer serve me with all the necessary tools to stay ahead of these ever-growing epidemic proportions of childhood disorders or dys-functions. Genetically modifying our food leads to the changing of its protein structures by adding other modified proteins. No one can control when they turn themselves on or off after they are part of the food. Here lies our biggest threat to our immune and digestive systems.

You may be asking yourself like me, how is it we have come to a place where those gifted and educated in medical research and organism design are involved in our food supply? Genetically modified organisms in pharmacology for the treatment of disease is certainly appropriate; but that same science used in the adaptation of our food puts us in nutritional jeopardy. It would then become a food (nutrition) that is not nutritious. How else can we explain what is taking place in our country in the last three decades? Over the years there has been a growing awareness of worsening and more complicated digestive challenges. They have brought on *Forceful terminologies*: Are we becoming more sophisticated or are our digestive needs becoming more aggressive? We used to call fungal problems "Candida" overgrowth but now it is Fungal Dysbiosis (overgrowth of mixed yeast in our foods) or how about Cerebral allergies (autism or anxiety)!

Our Children are suffering Epidemic proportions:

- Autism
- Allergies up 400% and effects one in four children
- Asthma up 300%
- ADHD up 400% and effects one in eleven children
- Gluten sensitivities/intolerances.
- Celiac disease
- Diabetes
- Eosinophilic Gastritis (unable to break down all food)
- Early onset menopause or andropause
- Obesity; 79.2% of Americans are obese yet many show signs of malnutrition.
- Toxins are now discovered in infant formulas
- Emergency room visits for food allergies are up and doubling each year

Genetic engineering in modern agricultural technology has now modified our food sources beyond what our human digestive system can recognize or our immune systems can defend. Manipulated opportunistic microorganisms or molecular proteins added into our food sources—whether to lessen caloric intake or to protect our crops may be the origin of our problems. Keep in mind most of our immune system can be found in our digestive tract along with the body's inflammatory responses.

"Scientists ... have detected the insecticidal protein ... circulating in the blood of pregnant as well as non-pregnant women. They have also detected the toxin in fetal blood, implying it could pass on to the next generation." In case it's not clear, I want to reiterate that this new study in Reproductive Technology has confirmed that if you eat GMO foods that contain the insecticidal BT toxin, it appears that it will be transferred to your bloodstream. As of now, about 90 percent of the corn grown in the United States is genetically engineered to either produce an insecticide, or to survive the application of herbicide. In addition, about 91-93 percent of all soybeans are genetically engineered to survive massive doses of Roundup herbicide. What this means is that nearly ALL foods you buy that contain either corn or soy, in any form, will contain GMO components unless certified organic by the USDA.

Again, the only way you can tell that you are not eating them is if the food has a green organic seal. Raw fruit and vegetables are marked organic or have numbers on their package that start with the number 9 on their label. If its numbers start with 3 or 4, they are grown on GMO soil, and the number 8 means they are totally GMO. Most of the foods that are canned, boxed, or bagged generally contain GMOs. Grass-fed beef; hormone-free poultry and eggs will be marked organic or free of GMOs. We used to feel safe when eating fresh wild fish and then they came up with the genetically-modified salmon.

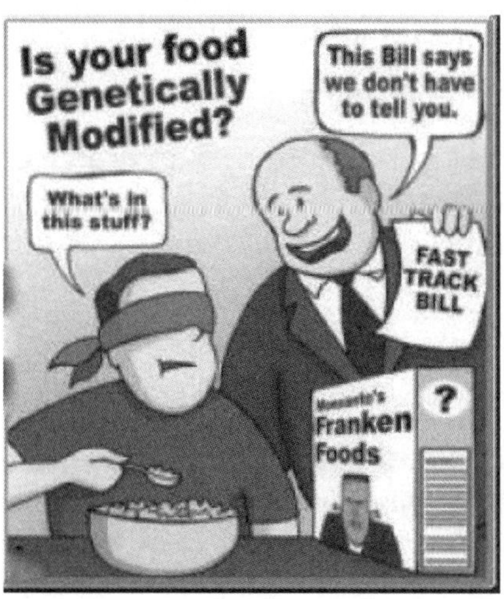
Is your food Genetically Modified?
This Bill says we don't have to tell you.
What's in this stuff?
FAST TRACK BILL
Franken Foods
?

Sometimes GMOs are referred to as "Franken Foods" and demands that we become educated in telling the difference in food which is no longer nutritious. We are left to deal with the consequences! What can we do if I may ask? I am suggesting that everyone have this foundational package included below at their home: Babies to adults can take these supplements without problems as long as they do not contain fillers or additives. Pregnant women and babies cannot take animal enzymes (pancreatin) because of the additives necessary to protect them from the stomach. Everyone should take:

- Supplemental plant-based **Digestive enzymes** ingested with every meal.
- Gluten sensitive people need a product that is formulated for this need.
- Supplemental plant-based **Protease enzymes** ingested between meals for immune balance and clearing the system of unrecognized proteins, biofilm, or fibrin.
- **Probiotics** taken before bed to recapture our healthy gut microorganisms and rid the system of opportunistic bacteria.

Just to show you how serious and yet ridiculous this has become, I list just a few of the engineered foods in which they received money from our government in grants and are given patents.

Scientists have worked on some thought-provoking combinations:

- Spider genes were inserted into goat DNA, in hopes that the goat milk would contain spider web protein for use in bulletproof vests.
- Cow genes turned pigskins into cowhides.
- Jellyfish genes lit up pigs' noses in the dark.
- Arctic fish genes gave tomatoes and strawberries tolerance to frost.
- Potatoes that glowed in the dark when they needed watering.
- Human genes were inserted into corn to produce spermicide.

Current field trials include:

- Corn engineered with human genes (Dow)
- Sugar cane engineered with human genes (Hawaii Agriculture Research Center)
- Corn engineered with jellyfish genes (Stanford University)
- Tobacco engineered with lettuce genes (University of Hawaii)

- Rice engineered with human genes (Applied Phytologics)
- Corn engineered with hepatitis virus genes (Prodigene)

"We all walk in the dark and each of us must learn to turn on his or her own light"
- Earl Nightingale

It is bad enough that we have genetically modified organisms in our food that our bodies do not recognize; but consider the added sugar for better taste = added toxicity at our cells, which spells disease.

If you are among those whose brain chemistry, taste buds, and hormones have been taken over by the food industry (up to 70 percent of us, including 40 percent of children), then it is time to stop blaming yourself and consider your own food rehab or a sugar detox. It is time for all of us to take back our health and demand that our children be protected from addictive substances in our schools and from the insidious marketing practices directed at them from the food industry.

DO YOU CRAVE SUGAR?

Crave means to long for, yearn for, hunger for, thirst for, set one's heart on, be bent on, desire, want, wish for, sigh for, pine for, lust after, covet, etc.

I will ask the question again...do you crave sugar? Most of us have felt the urge or unstoppable craving to look for something sweet when we are losing energy as we do mid-afternoon. What is it we look for to give us a pick up? Have you ever made a decision to allow no sweets in the house and then tear the house apart looking for something—anything sweet to devour. That uncontrollable hunger for sweets even though you know it will make you fat or sick.

SUGAR IS A HARDWIRED BRAIN RESPONSE

This craving or absolute need for sweets is now being proved that it is a powerful hardwired brain response over which we feel we have little control. At a restaurant many times you find yourself facing a basket of bread that you want to tear into and consume all of it before the entrée is served. How many times have we asked for another basket be brought to the table even before our appetizer is served.

SAD (STANDARD AMERICAN DIET)

Debate has raged recently about whether junk food, the hyper-processed, hyper-palatable food that has become our SAD (Standard American Diet) is addictive in the same way that heroin or cocaine is addictive. A new study published in the

American Journal of Clinical Nutrition suggests that, in fact, higher sugar, higher glycemic foods can be addictive.

David Ludwig, author of *Ending the Food Fight*, and his colleagues at Harvard, in a very sophisticated study, showed that foods with more sugar—foods that raise blood sugar even more than table sugar such as white flour, white potatoes, and refined starch have what is called a high-glycemic index—trigger a special region in the brain called the nucleus accumbens which is known as the area of our brain for reward, pleasure, reinforcement learning, addiction, aggression, fear, and impulsivity. It is known for addictions such as gambling or drug abuse.

Their theory is strong since it appears part of the reason almost 70 percent of Americans are overweight or one in two Americans has Type 2 diabetes may not be gluttony, lack of willpower, or absence of personal responsibility, but plain old garden variety biological addiction.

PLEASURE AND REINFORCEMENT

Many previous studies have shown how this region of brain, the pleasure center, lights up in response to emotionally arousing pictures, sexual images, even images of eating sugary, processed, or junk food. But this new study actually took on the hard job of proving the biology of sugar addiction. The researchers did a randomized, blinded, crossover study using the most rigorous research design to ward off any criticism. They took 12 overweight or obese men between the ages of 18 and 35 and gave each a low sugar or low glycemic index (37 percent) milkshake, and then, four hours later, they measured the activity of the brain region (*nucleus accumbency*) that controls addiction. They also measured blood sugar and hunger.

Then, days later they had them back for another milkshake. But this time they switched the milkshakes. They were designed to taste exactly the same and be exactly the same in every way except in how much and how quickly it spiked blood sugar. The second milkshake was designed to be high in sugar with a high glycemic index (84 percent). The shakes had exactly the same amount of calories, protein, fat, and carbohydrate. The participants didn't know which milkshake they were getting, and their mouth couldn't tell the difference, but their brains could.

Each participant received a brain scan and blood tests for glucose and insulin after each version of the milkshake. They were their own control group. Without exception, they all had the same response. The high sugar or glycemic index milkshake caused a spike in blood sugar and insulin and an increase in reported hunger and cravings four hours after the shake. Remember — exactly the same calories, sweetness, texture, and macronutrient content. But the breakthrough finding was this: When the high-glycemic shake was consumed, the *nucleus accumbens* lit up like a Christmas tree. This pattern occurred in every single participant and was statistically significant.

This study showed two things:

- First, the body responds quite differently to different calories, even if the protein, fat, and carbs (and taste) are exactly the same.
- Second, foods that spike blood sugar are biologically addictive.

This game-changing study must force a shift in the conversation about obesity in America. There are 600,000 processed foods in the marketplace, 80 percent of which have added hidden sugar. The average American consumes 22 teaspoons of mostly hidden sugar, and the average teenage boy has 34 teaspoons a day (more than two 20-ounce sodas). One serving of Prego tomato sauce has more sugar than a serving of Oreo cookies. Sweetened yogurts can have more sugar than a can of soda. Read the carbohydrate count of foods and then the actual sugar count. You may see that the sugar may be switched with synthetic sugars and you might think this is best. The synthetic sugar has a taste that is anywhere from 400 to 600 times sweeter. Their use is more of a disease-forming problem, or at least as much as sugar.

Sugar is the core ingredient used by the food industry to make bad ingredients (processed flour and chemicals) taste good. Our consumption has increased from when sugar cane was introduced years ago by the Jesuit missionaries in the late 1700s to a producer of sugar here in the United States, based in Florida, which produces 700,000 tons of raw sugar annually. They have the newest cane sugar refinery in the US. What went from sucking on a sugar cane to the average American consuming 140 pounds of sugar a year and also consuming 133 pounds of white or wheat flour, which raises blood sugar more than table sugar (sucrose).

No one wants to be fat or become a drug addict. No one wants their life destroyed by disability and illness. We have policies and laws that protect people from alcohol, tobacco and illegal drugs of abuse. Sugar and flour (and too much starchy white potatoes and white rice) or products containing them appear to be no different. In fact, some animal studies show that sugar is eight times as addictive as cocaine.

It is time to stop blaming the uneducated fat person. Can we really blame our children if we freely give them drugs of abuse in the school lunch line or as after-school snacks? Can we really blame the average overweight person? The nutritional landscape in America is a food carnival.

Kelly Brownell from Yale's Rudd Center for Food Policy and Obesity has created a validated food questionnaire to help you determine if you are a food addict. He recently also published a textbook, *Food and Addiction*, that lays out the science of how our hyper-processed, hyper-palatable, hyper-sweet industrial food has hijacked our brain chemistry and biology.

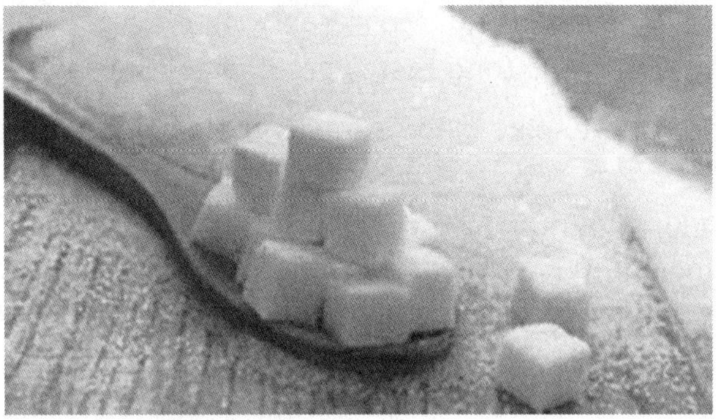

Here are five clues you may be addicted to sugar, flour, and processed food. Ask yourself if you can answer yes to each of these questions:

- You consume certain foods even if you are not hungry because of cravings.
- You worry about cutting down on certain foods.
- You feel sluggish or fatigued from overeating.
- You have health or social problems (affecting school or work) because of food issues and yet keep eating the way you do despite negative consequences.
- You need more and more of the foods you crave to experience any pleasure or reduce negative emotions.

Chapter 8

Enhance Your Mental Capacity by Your Digestive System

Our brain is considered as our second gut or you could say our digestive system is our second brain. Isn't it interesting that we constantly use the term "my gut-feeling tells me"?

THINK OF YOUR GUT AS YOUR SECOND BRAIN

Actually, you have two brains, one inside your skull and one in your gut, and each needs its own vital nourishment. Your gut and brain actually work in tandem, each influencing the other. This is why your intestinal health can have such a profound influence on your mental health, and vice versa; as well as the reason why your diet is so closely linked to your mental health. According to research, probiotics have a significant effect on brain chemistry, modulating mood and behavior, regulating signals to your brain via the vagus nerve.

You may not be aware that you actually have two nervous systems: central nervous system composed of your brain and spinal cord and the enteric nervous system, which is the intrinsic nervous system of your gastrointestinal tract that runs from your mouth to your anus.

Both are actually created out of the same type of tissue. During fetal development, one part turns into your central nervous system while the other develops into your enteric nervous system. These two systems are connected via the vagus nerve; the tenth cranial nerve that runs from your brain stem down to your abdomen. It is now well established that the vagus nerve is indeed the primary route your gut bacteria use to transmit information to your brain.

The brain exchange center of the nervous system is where sensations generate ideas, and ideas are expressed by action. Evidence of its importance to the body comes from the fact that the brain accounts for only two percent of the body's weight; yet its operation uses 20 percent of the oxygen and blood. It is a mass of soft, spongy, pinkish-gray nerve tissue. The weight of the brain in an average adult is about three pounds. The neurons, or nerve cell bodies, fit together as precisely and compactly as a puzzle. They are so intimately coordinated as to allow the size and shape of the brain to be used to maximum efficiency.

Neither the weight nor the size of the brain is a reliable clue to the intelligence of the individual. The size of the cells does not matter, either; rather, the number of brain cells is exceedingly important. The human brain, and that of higher animals, is not fully formed at birth. Like life itself, the brain is a growing, flowing thing. It first becomes discernible in the human embryo about two weeks after conception. A thin, gray film of cortex begins to spread across its upper surface. It crinkles as growth continues and it nestles into the cerebrum. At birth, the human baby is about one-third head and literally top-heavy with brains. The infant brain is still only an overgrown seed, weighing in at only 25 percent of its adult weight. Just as muscles grow with exercise, so does the brain as the child gets older and uses the brain's countless parts and pathways. The structure of the brain is formed by the mental experiences of the growing child. This formation is the most rapid in the preschool years. However, it continues to a lesser degree throughout life. About 50 percent of the brain's capacity is genetically inherited, while the other 50 percent is culturally shaped (by teaching and example). Day by day, the living brain models itself biologically as a physical organ. Language, images, and ideas continually course through its convoluted passages. The brain is protected from harmful substances in the bloodstream by the blood-brain barrier. It keeps most toxins away from the brain, or at least delays their entry for several hours, sometimes days. If the toxins have already penetrated other parts of the body, they are blocked from the brain.

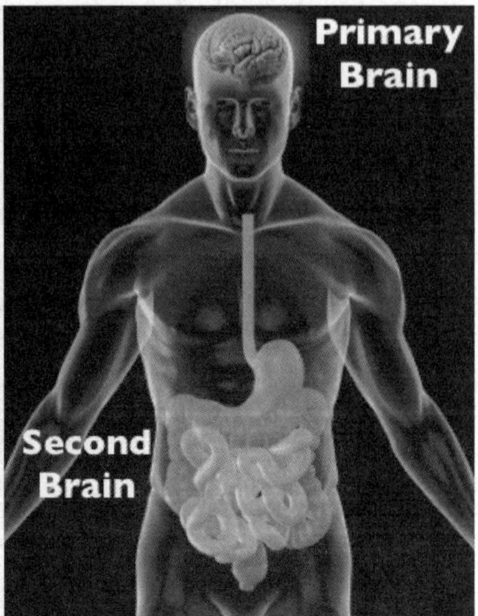

The hypothalamus, an organ the size of a lump of sugar, is located at the base of the cerebrum (the upper, main part of the brain, consisting of the left and right hemispheres). Although it is very small, the hypothalamus controls some very vital functions, including the ebb and flow of the body's fluids, the regulation of fat and carbohydrate metabolism, blood sugar levels, and body temperature. It directs the rhythmic cycles, such as activity and rest, appetite and digestion, sexual desire, and the menstrual and reproductive functions. In addition, the hypothalamus is the body's "emotional" brain. This miraculous little organ is the coordinating center for the nervous system. It controls our sleep, wakefulness, alertness, and reactions to pain and pleasure. Without this gland, I would not be writing this book if everything I discuss here depends on the hypothalamus! The question then arises – how does the hypothalamus receive its information?

Think Twice: How the Gut's 'Second Brain' Influences Mood and Well-Being. *The emerging and surprising view of how the enteric nervous system in our digestive tract goes far beyond just processing the food we eat.*

A deeper understanding of this mass of neural tissue, filled with important neurotransmitters, is revealing that it does much more than merely handle digestion or inflict the occasional nervous pang. The little brain in our gut, in connection with the big one in our skulls, partly determines our mental state and plays key roles in certain diseases throughout the body.

Although its influence is far-reaching, the second brain is not the seat of any conscious thoughts or decision-making.

"The second brain doesn't help with the great thought processes...religion, philosophy, and poetry is left to the brain in the head," says Dr. Michael Gershon of Columbia University Medical Center.

Technically known as the enteric nervous system, the second brain consists of sheaths of neurons embedded in the walls of the long tube of our digestive system, or alimentary canal, which measures about nine meters end to end from the esophagus to the anus.

The second brain contains some 100 million neurons, more than in either the spinal cord or the peripheral nervous system.

This multitude of neurons in the enteric nervous system enables us to "feel" the inner world of our gut and its contents. Much of this neural firepower comes to bear in the elaborate daily grind of digestion. Breaking down food, absorbing nutrients, and expelling of waste require chemical processing, mechanical mixing, and rhythmic muscle contractions that move everything on down the line.

Thus equipped with its own reflexes and senses, the second brain can control gut behavior independently of the brain. We likely evolved this intricate web of nerves to perform digestion and excretion "on site," rather than remotely from our brains through the middleman of the spinal cord. "The brain in the head doesn't need to get its hands dirty with the messy business of digestion, which is delegated to the brain in the gut!" says Gershon. However, the second brain's complexity likely cannot be interpreted through this process alone.

"The system is way too complicated to have evolved only to make sure things move out of your colon," states UCLA professor Emeran Mayer. For example, scientists were shocked to learn that about 90 percent of the fibers in the primary visceral nerve, the vagus, carry information from the gut to the brain and not the other way around. "Some of that info is decidedly unpleasant," says Gershon.

The second brain informs our state of mind in other ways, as well. "A big part of our emotions are probably influenced by the nerves in our gut," says Mayer. Butterflies in the stomach, signaling in the gut as part of our physiological stress response, is but one example. Although gastrointestinal (GI) turmoil can sour one's mood, everyday emotional well-being may rely on messages from the brain below to the brain above. For example, electrical stimulation of the vagus nerve—a useful treatment for depression—may mimic these signals.

Given the two brains' commonalities, other depression treatments that target the mind can unintentionally impact the gut. The enteric nervous system uses more than 30 neurotransmitters, just like the brain, and in fact 95 percent of the body's serotonin is found in the bowels.

Because antidepressant medications called selective serotonin reuptake inhibitors (SSRIs) increase serotonin levels, it's little wonder that meds meant to cause chemical changes in the mind often provoke GI issues as a side effect. Irritable bowel syndrome, which afflicts more than two million Americans, also arises in part from too much serotonin in our gut, and could perhaps be regarded as a "mental illness" of the second brain.

Scientists are learning that the serotonin made by the enteric nervous system might also play a role in more surprising diseases: In a new Nature Medicine study published online February 7, 2014, a drug that inhibited the release of serotonin from the gut counteracted the bone-deteriorating disease osteoporosis in postmenopausal rodents.

Serotonin seeping from the second brain might even play some part in autism, the developmental disorder often first noticed in early childhood. Gershon has discovered that the same genes involved in synapse formation between neurons in the brain are involved in the alimentary synapse formation. "If these genes are affected in autism," he says, "it could explain why so many kids with autism have GI motor abnormalities," in addition to elevated levels of gut-produced serotonin in their blood.

Down the road, the blossoming field of Neurogastroenterology will likely offer some new insight into the workings of the second brain and its impact on the body and mind. "We have never systematically looked at [the enteric nervous system] in relating lesions in it to diseases like they have for the" central nervous system. One day, perhaps there will be well-known connections between diseases and lesions in the gut's nervous system as some in the brain and spinal cord today indicate multiple sclerosis.

Cutting-edge research is currently investigating how the second brain mediates the body's immune response; after all, at least 80 percent of our immune system is aimed at the gut to expel and kill foreign invaders.

Mayer is doing work on how the trillions of bacteria in the gut "communicate" with enteric nervous system cells (which they greatly outnumber). His work with the gut's nervous system has led him to think that in coming years psychiatry will need to expand to the brain in the gut.

Now, I will take a look at the connection between the second brain and the body, and how supplemental digestive plant-based enzymes support them. Food is defined as anything ingested into the body that serves to nourish or build tissues and cells. The book titled *Brain Allergies* (published by Keats Publishing Inc., copyright 1980) by Doctors William H. Philpoot, M.D., and Dwight K. Kalita, Ph.D, states: "A person cannot be nutritionally deficient, toxic, infected, or addicted to any food or chemical without suffering the consequences of progression of the disease process into a chronic degenerative illness of some type."

Previous studies have already linked sugary drinks with a host of diseases including obesity, diabetes, high blood pressure, high cholesterol, cancer, coronary artery disease, and gout.

"Soda remains the largest source of added sugar in the diet," Dr. Adam Bernstein, study author and Research Director at Cleveland Clinic's Wellness Institute, said in a press release. "What we're beginning to understand is that regular intake of these beverages sets off a chain reaction in the second brain that can potentially lead to many diseases, including stroke." Researchers speculate that the high amount of sugar in sodas leads to rapid increases in blood glucose and insulin. These increase eventually to cause glucose intolerance, insulin resistance, and inflammation, which in turn influence the development of atherosclerosis and blood clots, and the stability of plaque.

The study, which was published in the American Journal of Clinical Nutrition, examined the soda intake of 43,371 men and 84,085 women and found that study participants who drank more than one soda daily had higher rates of blood pressure and blood cholesterol combined with lower rates of physical activity. The news was not any better for those who drank diet soda: They had a higher incidence of chronic disease and a higher body mass index (BMI).

Researchers found that sugary sodas increased the risk of ischemic stroke, caused when a blood vessel that supplies blood to the brain is blocked by a blood clot. Diet sodas fared no better, increasing the risk of hemorrhagic stroke, triggered when a weakened blood vessel bursts and causes hemorrhaging inside the brain. The risk for both types of stroke was higher in women compared to men.

It is vital to feed and fortify the second brain in order to have a healthy, balanced body. Many uninformed people will naturally assume this means eating sugar to energize the system. The media and other sources have conditioned us for years, all of them telling us to eat a candy bar or drink a cola beverage for that boost around three o'clock in the afternoon. However, brain food must be highly nutritional and must contain high levels of oxygen. If we have digestive and assimilation difficulties, both brains will suffer. When food remnants in the bloodstream reach the first brain, the barrier regards them as invaders. The hypothalamus operates our endocrine and nervous system, our two major control centers. It stands to reason that we should feed our brains only with the healthiest foods.

ENHANCE YOUR MENTAL CAPACITY

CASE HISTORY

One day a woman brought her husband to my office, a gentleman in his sixties. His son, a medical doctor, had tested him for Alzheimer's hoping to find a natural way to treat him; they requested diet and enzyme counseling from me. I suggested a diet suitable for his body type and enzyme formulations to feed and fortify his system. Keep in mind there is a time to feed and fortify and a time to detoxify. However, the beauty of enzymes is that these formulations allow us to do both at the same time and in harmony. I put him on a vigorous supplemental digestive enzymes and food plan, and they departed for their home in another state. Three weeks later, I received a phone call, followed by a letter. The elated wife told me that before beginning his enzyme program, her husband could not remember their children's names and could no longer read or watch television. After only a few weeks on enzymes, her husband wrote notes to her and was watching TV again. Within nine weeks, he was almost completely restored to his former self. Is this a miracle? Yes . . . it is the miracle of enzymes delivering nutrients to a depleted system that desperately needed them and in tandem, influencing the brain!

FIBROMYALGIA

FM is a "chronic invisible illness." It is not just a form of muscular rheumatism. It is actually a type of neurotransmitter dysfunction. One symptom is poor concentration. Exactly what is the nervous system and how does it affect our concentration? It is composed of the brain, the spinal cord, and the enteric nervous system. Collectively, these work in harmony with one another and serve as the communication and coordination systems of the body. The nervous system transports information to the brain and relays instructions from it. There are two subsystems that together could perform functions that are more complicated. The first is the autonomic nervous system. The caretaker of the body, it operates without conscious control, taking care of involuntary actions like breathing or the heartbeat. The voluntary nervous system includes both motor and sensory nerves. Among many other tasks, it controls our voluntary muscle movement and carries information to the brain. The command centers of both these systems lie in the hypothalamus. They are in perpetual activity, fine-tuning the body's processes to all the internal and external demands made upon it. Research is showing that people with FM have defects in the neuroregulatory system, especially transmitters and poor digestion that affects the brain neurotransmitters.

You should now understand that our enteric nervous system (second brain) runs throughout the digestive tract. You have heard many times that it is not a good idea to eat when you are upset, or if you have suffered severe trauma. When the body is stressed, many reactions are set into motion. Elevated levels of epinephrine are released into the blood to enhance muscle action. The liver immediately dispatches glucose, which is a source of instant energy for all the muscles. Heart rate and breathing accelerate, but digestive activity slows. Blood vessels constrict to cause sweating, so the body will stay cool while under stress. Now, the body is ready for some extraordinary actions.

While all this is taking place, the parasympathetic nervous system prevents these processes from speeding up to extreme rates. The parasympathetic, part of the autonomic system, originates in the midbrain. It monitors constriction of the eye pupils, slows the heartbeat, and stimulates certain digestive glands. The parasympathetic acts as a damper. If the trauma is not too serious, it allows the body to return to normal. It does not work as fast as the sympathetic system (also part of the autonomic system, which works in opposition to the parasympathetic, i.e., dilates the pupils, etc.). Messages from the brain, often in response to information conveyed by the sensory nerves, are delivered to the muscles by motor nerves. One motor nerve with its branching tendrils may control thousands of the muscle fibers.

All the parts of the nervous system are constantly interacting with one another. They are so well coordinated you can simultaneously think, feel, and act on many levels without confusion. We suffer neurological disorders if the organs of the nervous system are inflamed or affected by disease or injury. This manifest such as paralysis, seizures, or sensor malfunctions immediately happens. When we say we are nervous, it simply means we are in a state of excitability with great mental and physical unrest.

The foods we eat and the enzymes carrying the nutrients feed our nervous system. The enzyme action is what helps the nerves communicate with each other. Inflammation creates problems for the nervous system, the symptoms for which can be tenderness, pain, or paralysis of a limb. Toxic substances poison our nerves. Alcohol and any vitamin deficiency are the worst offenders. Diabetes poses additional difficulties for those with nervous disorders. Any type of allergy, as well as some viral or bacterial infections, has an impact on the nervous system.

Rest, therapeutic digestive enzymes, and a nutritious diet are the best treatments for these conditions. Extra vitamins from the B group are essential. However, they cannot be delivered without enzymes. Very few of the vitamin tablets on the market are chemical-free and can only be used by one half of the measured milligrams. Even enzymes cannot deliver the unused artificial compounds.

Foods called super foods, those highly nourishing ones that occur naturally, are those whose nutrients will actually be delivered. Chemical-made vitamins usually create more toxicity rather than provide any nutritional benefits. So if you take vitamins long term, make sure they are natural complex vitamins, not synthetics. For example, B6, B12, etc., should say Whole B Complex, not cutout with a chemical and measured as in B6–50mg. The absolute best are those freeze-dried vegetables that contain the truly natural synergy of the nutrients.

ANXIETY

Anxiety is a feeling of uneasiness, apprehension, or even dread. In many instances anxiety is a perfectly rational response. We may feel anxious about passing an exam at school, how well we will do at our new job, or moving to a new city. Realistic anxiety means we have pronounced concerns about world issues like war, the effects of toxic air, or social and economic conditions that affect our lifestyles. Our easy access to the mass media can serve to intensify normal anxieties. A certain amount of unrealistic and irrational anxiety is an accepted part of our daily lives.

Our awareness of both past and future can result in increased levels of anxiety during certain times of our lives, especially adolescence and middle age. People who spend much of their time alone are likely to suffer more anxiety than those who live and work with others. Most of us find healthy ways to work with our anxiety. We make new friends, take up new hobbies, become good listeners, and volunteer in our communities as a means of helping others. We can relieve our anxiety through exercise and physical activity. Games and sports, participating in group activities, or taking a good walk often dissipates an anxious mood. Real anxiety is created by something specific and identifiable, such as alcohol. When anxiety is chronic and not traceable to a specific cause, we call it neurosis. This is an especially difficult one, because it always interferes with normal activity. Often the sufferer is subject to extreme fear. It becomes pathological when the individual can no longer control his emotions. It may be severe enough to manifest as organic pain or true physical illness. The best way to fight anxiety is to find its cause. Identify your own specific body type and investigate your food allergies and choices. This will greatly help you to alleviate the problem.

ENERVATION: THE CAUSE OF ANXIETY AND NERVOUSNESS

Enervation is physically-induced anxiety. The word itself speaks of being drained of energy or fatigue. We can enervate ourselves in a variety of ways. Overeating, too much alcohol, sugar, cooked food, salt, caffeine, tobacco, drugs, and impure water consumption, as well as over-work, worry, tension, depression, and lack of rest all serve to enervate us. When these habits are dropped, headaches and general letdown usually occur. As the body discards toxins, it is normal to experience depression, a decrease in energy and feeling generally unwell. You have heard the expressions, "You need to feel bad to feel good," or "You will get a lot sicker before you get better." Several times when treating clients, I have found that these beliefs have kept them from giving me an accurate picture of their health. They assume they should feel unwell, and it is not important enough to let me know about it. After realizing what was happening, I could match the enzymes with their needs. This fortified their bodies, creating a greater sense of well-being and increased stamina. I believe a great deal of the disease we see in our society today is caused by enervation. Enervation resides in almost every home in the country.

Years ago when I first began my practice in nutrition, the first two weeks of association with a new client required great vigilance on my part. During those times, the client was in desperate need for motivation. Many of them were, at first, under the false impression that they did better on junk foods. It was my responsibility to get them through the first stages of withdrawal. I heard complaints of weakness, of feeling a lack in the necessary strength to continue. Often the weakness and the results of the dietary changes were blamed on me! I had to do some fancy footwork to convince them of the need for "house cleaning." Sometimes it was very difficult to accept the fact that it was normal to feel ill. The more toxic the body, the worse they felt.

Now, I realize when a client is experiencing cleansing and still feels ill and fatigued, it is because I did not match the correct amount of supplemental plant-based enzymes to their needs. The body will move through a catabolic state. It rids itself of old obstructive material that has been stored in the tissue and joints. However, when we ingest the correct amount of foods high in nutritional value, renewed strength and rejuvenation occur.

I like to see each client two weeks after the initial visit. I know the client will be in a recuperative period and that the enzymes will have done a good part of their work. Most of the clients' education takes place at the second visit. Frequently, they have more questions about diet. This establishes a working knowledge between us of where we are in their wellness cycle. One month later, I see them a third time. Where they are now in an anabolic (constructive metabolism—the process by which food is changed into living tissue) stage of healthy living. From time to time, as you continue to build good health, you may experience common cold or other symptoms. If this occurs, simply return to the routine initially prescribed for the enzymes. This type of recurrence is usually due to not taking the correct quantity of protease while detoxifying. I am very committed to the principle that the more clients are educated and encouraged, the more likely they will take responsibility for their own progress. I have an open-door policy. I always want my clients to feel free to ask questions about their healing and their state of balance.

As a teacher in the field of building good health, I have discovered I must have patience, thoroughness, and kindness. These are easily recognized traits. If they are not found, the prospective client will go elsewhere. This does not mean the he can get away without assuming any responsibility for himself. When I think of someone about to undertake a natural health regimen, it brings two old adages to mind: *"You can lead a horse to water, but you can't make him drink,"* and *"There are no incurable diseases; there are only incurable people."*

Prospective clients come to me after they have doctored themselves for years by taking various medications. Yet, they are still miserable and sick and never really feel good. When they hear about the enzyme program, they expect to feel like new overnight. That will not happen. You must be very committed anytime you decide that you are going to start a new, healthy lifestyle. If the program is going to work, it will not be a fad or trendy diet. Rather, it will be tailored to your needs and your body type. You cannot change your body type, who you are, what your family is like, your strengths and weaknesses by simply changing your mind. Some things we bring into our lives are hereditary. As we get closer to a balanced state, it may be more difficult to recognize our body type. I ask each client to take the enzymes for at least three to nine weeks from the initial visit. As they progress, I will move them into a maintenance program.

Education begins when enervation (fatigue or exhaustion) is detected. Rebuilding a consciousness of wellness is a good starting point. People who suffer from anxiety often forget to breathe! Since oxygenating the blood is critical to good health, it is no wonder so many of us feels ill and fatigued all the time. The purpose of breathing is to supply oxygen to the body and to aid in cleansing the blood stream. Breath is life. It has been said that we learn to breathe a few seconds after we are born, and when we forget to breathe, we die. Abnormal cells multiply in the absence of oxygen. The significance of proper breathing and fresh air cannot be over-emphasized. Some have a problem of breathing because of an acid/alkaline imbalance caused by poor food choices for their own unique body types.

What happens when we breathe? The chest rises and falls while the diaphragm expands and contracts. This naturally creates a vacuum into which air rushes. Finally, the air is forced from the lungs. Blood then enters the lungs to pick up the oxygen and carry it to the cells. At the same time, it takes on carbon dioxide that has been expelled by the cells. The entire process is automatically controlled. This respiratory center is located in the medulla oblongata at the base of the brain where the top of the spinal cord widens. Carbon dioxide acts as a stimulant of the respiratory center. The more carbon dioxide present in the blood, the more the respiratory center is stimulated and the faster we breathe. Conversely, the more oxygen in the blood, the slower we breathe because oxygen inhibits the medulla. Our breath rate and volume are adjusted constantly to the body's need at every single moment. If the air around us is clean, it gives us energy. I encourage everyone to spend time outdoors, breathing fresh air as much as possible since we are living beings and breath is life.

I closely observe people as they relate their stories of illness to me. Many times they rush through these tales, never stopping to breathe. It is sad to me how our society has become so anxiety-ridden. May I say again, the way to make a change is to make a change! Do the things you find pleasurable. To go beyond exhaustion, we must change the way we eat and change our attitude.

ATTITUDE

I will never stop saying how crucial it is for you to develop a good, positive attitude. This is of extreme importance in the practice of good health. Remember, there are no incurable diseases; there are only incurable people. I know people who would rather sit around all day and talk about their illnesses than do anything about them. Why do this? Their thinking is misguided. They are self-absorbed and negative because of self-poisoning and thus allowing them to be brainwashed into thinking ill health is normal. We discuss our health in everyday conversation as much as we talk about the weather. Ever since the days of Freud, we have been taught to cure our problems by dwelling on them. The efforts of psychiatrists and psychologists today help to perpetuate this, leaving us with uncured mental health maladies and a prevailing order of failure and chaos. There is an above-average rate of suicide among these mental health practitioners. Dr. Abraham Maslow, a brilliant psychologist, has changed all that. He said, "What we need is a new direction. We ought to stop dwelling on the sick and the deranged if we want to restore people to a perfect mental health.

We ought to study health; not illness. We ought not to treat illness but to direct the person into the life patterns of the mentally healthy." Those who are using Dr. Maslow's philosophy are revolutionizing the mental health field with tremendous results. I have found it is far more effective to talk about healthy knuckles, rather than the arthritis afflicting a client's hands.

Those who are truly successful in building optimum health are those who never look back once they have established healthy new life patterns. They focus on constant rejuvenation of the body's systems. The food you eat is your body's fuel. These foods nourish and fortify our nervous and endocrine systems with healthy nutrients. I ask you to remember at all times, we cannot take synthetic, chemical vitamins and expect them to be delivered to our cells. The body is not designed to assimilate chemicals. It will attempt to digest and deliver them, but in the process it uses up precious metabolic enzymes needed to rebuild nerves and tissues. Plant-based enzymes will only deliver pure, natural nutrients. Common sense tells us these nutrients should come from one source: pure, natural foods. If you want to nourish your nerves and your immune and endocrine systems, you must ingest a certain amount of protein, complex carbohydrates, and some fats. Our nerve fibers are made of protein and fat.

BANISHING HEADACHE PAIN

A pain or ache in the head . . . I have a headache! The headache is one of the most common ailments known to humanity. Most of us do not know that it is actually a symptom rather than a disorder in itself. We all are familiar with it. It may come as a stab between the eyes when you eat cold food too quickly. Perhaps it is the ever-tightening clamp of tense muscles around your head. Worst of all, it can be the "lock me in a dark room until it's over" pain of a migraine. If you suffer from a headache, you treat it as most of us do. We either wait for it to stop or go for the bewildering array of pain medications over-the-counter. Often, this is sufficient treatment. However if you have a headache more than three times a month, you need to take a close look at the possible causes. It is reported that recurrent migraine or tension type headaches are seen in about 50 percent of FM patients.

There are three types of headaches. The first, a tension headache, is that tightening band of pressure around your head. This is triggered by stress and usually lasts anywhere from 30 minutes to seven days. In the worst cases, it lasts all day every day. Cluster headaches cause excruciating pain behind or around one eye. Sometimes this pain radiates into the temple, jaw, nose, chin, or teeth. Nasal congestion, sweating, watery eyes, and a flushed face can add to the discomfort. This type of headache may occur three times in a day, lasting from 15 to 90 minutes for up to 16 weeks at a time. Migraines bring on severe, pulsating pain, nausea, and sensitivity to light and noise. Many migraine sufferers retire to a darkened room until the pain subsides. This can take anywhere from two hours to three days.

Medical doctors urge patients with serious headaches to keep a headache diary. It is very helpful to record the intensity, duration, symptoms, the degree to which the patient is disabled, and how he is affected by any prescribed treatments. The doctors may even recommend fighting headaches with changes in eating, sleep, or work habits. Other treatments used commonly are physical therapy, biofeedback, and drugs. For tension headaches, physical therapy, hot packs, cold packs, or electrical stimulation devices such as ultrasound and massage are the accepted treatments. Biofeedback helps about 80 percent of the time, and it is the only non-pharmaceutical treatment that works for migraines. It is somewhat helpful for tension headaches, but completely ineffective for cluster headaches.

The most common causes of a headache:

Allergies	Sinus Infection	Hunger	Arthritis
Red Wines	Head Trauma	Blood Pressure	Hangover
Caffeine Withdrawal	Disease	Cold or Flu	TMJ Disorder
Food	Eyestrain		

Foods that cause most of our headaches are aged cheeses, smoked meats, chocolate, alcohol (especially red wines), homemade yeast breads, raisins, avocados, and MSG, an additive in Chinese and processed foods.

Those who suffer from chronic headache are usually in a state of enervation. Their lifestyles and diets do not work for them, so they experience headache interference. This indicates it is time to make changes. Often it is a change in food choices that works the best. The support products used in my practice make healing the headache a simple process. I am thrilled to see the amazing properties of enzymes doing the work for which nature intended them. My experience with headache treatment through the use of enzyme therapy is always the same. The headaches become a thing of the past, even those intense migraines.

When I meet a client for the first time, I cannot always know what causes the headache because many different factors are involved. No matter what the cause, I begin with protease in order to create a healthier immune system. Dosages of 330,000 to over 400,000 units of activity several times daily are initially required to make a difference with those who have toxic undigested foods in the bloodstream. One of the products I formulated includes herbs to feed and fortify the nervous system. Other herbs are used as antioxidants that add oxygen to the blood. When these two specific formulas are used together, protease and the herbal compound, the results are stunning. I conclude from this that most headaches are caused by one of two things. First, widespread toxicity in the body, sufficient to prevent the breakdown of food particles in the digestive tract, is a primary cause of headaches. Second, a stressful event taking place that involved the nervous or endocrine system also produces headaches. When I give either the protease or the herbs and enzymes combined, the headache frequently disappears within moments. After using this formulation for a short time, those migraine sufferers realize they are not having the headaches as often or as intensely as they once did. If the headaches come back, the client must readjust the care he is giving to himself and get right back on track. Keep in mind, a headache is a symptom indicating something is wrong in the body. It is not a disease itself.

It is important to remember that stress is not an external force. Developing from an internal source, it is the result of cellular contamination and nutritional deficiency. Manifestations of stress take the form of pain, fatigue, anxiety, disability, and malfunction. These are the direct results of substandard health conditions. The stress due to poor health can be light, mild, moderate, serious, and severe. If we are experiencing light stress, usually there will not be any kind of physical symptom to inform us of its occurrence. With mild stress, we may sometimes feel slightly out of sorts. In moderate stress constant symptoms are present, though they are still sufficiently weak to be merely annoying. Serious or severe stress will undoubtedly manifest in some way, often as strong pain. This is the body reacting to the stress of cellular contamination and nutritional deficiencies. It has finally reached the point where it can no longer endure the stresses imposed upon it without physical manifestations. The common response is, of course, to take some kind of therapy to alleviate the pain and other symptoms. This is certainly appropriate, but it does not address the cause of the problem. It is only a matter of time before the malfunction returns, possibly in the same form. However, it can be in a much more severe form or a totally different one. Looking at it as a healthcare professional, I believe an individual with health stress manifestations should be placed on a health-building program that complements the immediate therapy prescribed by his or her doctor. This would guarantee that the reasons for the stress are properly addressed.

The new choices offered for a health-building program would include foods appropriate for the client's body type and eliminate the ones that create stress. Plant-based supplemental enzymes will aid the digestion assimilation, utilization, and elimination of the food ingested. Protease will be taken to destroy cellular contaminants. Other enzyme fortifiers will eradicate nutritional deficiencies. Good health would return to the patient. No matter the symptom or problem, learn to change your habits for the better and return to a path that gives life to your system.

RECURRENT HEADACHES IN CHILDREN AND ADOLESCENTS

Our children are suffering from headaches that come up often. We are now recognizing that these children have long-term anxiety. Recurrent headaches defined as the occurrence of less than 15 days with headache/month, are common in children and adolescents (those under 20 years of age, referred to collectively as children). Who gets it? About 50 percent of seven year olds and almost 85 percent of 15 year olds report such headaches. Children, who are as young as two years of age, can also complain of headaches. Boys and girls are equally affected. Girls may be more affected when compared to boys in their late teens. These headaches from anxiety many times keep these children home from school and from having an active life.

STRESS AND HYPERTENSION: CALMING YOUR NERVES AND REDUCING ANXIETY

The best example to demonstrate the interdependence of the body's many systems is the nervous system. Earlier in this chapter, I characterized the endocrine and nervous systems as the two major control centers. We know the hormones cannot function without a strong and well-balanced endocrine system. Consider that the nerves, like the hormones, are closely related to the endocrine system. One of the physiological responses created by the electrical impulses from the nerves is the secretion of hormones by the endocrine glands. Yet, the nervous system receives its support from the endocrine system. Research shows that people with Fibromyalgia have low-growth hormone, which is involved with muscle repair.

The complexity of your nervous system is truly mind-boggling. Electrical impulses in the neuro-chemical process travel throughout your body. The system is a perfectly coordinated network of nerve cells—possibly in the hundreds of billions—that are tied to threadlike formations. These work together to process and respond to information from all your senses. When nerve cells die, they are not replaced; hence, an older person has many millions less than a youngster. If you suffer nerve damage, only a limited amount of repair is possible. The cells are obviously very sensitive and will not perform well if our brain is perturbed by a concentration of undigested protein fragments or a shortage of oxygen or glucose. All this begins to thicken the plot. Not only is a sufficient supply of enzymes necessary to fortify and revitalize our endocrine system, which in turn supports our nerves, but those same enzymes are vital for complete digestion. The digestion is what allows our nerves to do their job.

Clients with anxiety problems often complain of other difficulties. In most cases, we can trace these back to the same fundamental cause—an overall bodily imbalance. The lack of internal equilibrium or challenged homeostasis is the true culprit. After a regimen of enzymes, calming herbs, and the appropriate genetic diet for his or her own specific body type, the client shows a dramatic improvement in both health and mental and emotional outlook.

HYPERTENSION

High blood pressure, or hypertension, can cause or aggravate disorders like heart attack, stroke, and kidney disease. Weight loss will significantly lower blood pressure without the use of drugs. A Journal of the American Medical Association study revealed that losing only eight pounds reduces diastolic (the reading taken when the heart muscle relaxes and the chambers fill with blood) blood pressure by an average of 2.3 points. Walking four or five times a week for 30 to 45 minutes will create an overall reduction of the blood pressure. Eating less salt, if you have a high blood reading, will lower diastolic blood pressure an average of one point as long as your blood sodium is high. Diastolic pressure is the second of two numbers in the blood pressure reading such as 137 over 80. Those with a reading of 90 or above have high blood pressure.

The findings of the American Medical Association showed that in spite of the widespread belief that emotional stress can elevate blood pressure, no benefit was gained from participating in a stress management program or taking vitamin supplements. Researchers from 11 medical centers are collaborating on an ongoing project sponsored by the National Heart, Lung and Blood Institute in Bethesda, Maryland. They are seeking ways to prevent high blood pressure from developing in people who face a higher-than-usual risk for it. A diet low in sodium and high in potassium helped, but not nearly so significantly as losing weight. The sodium concern has become more complicated recently. It depends on the sodium in your blood. Most doctors order this part of blood test. There have been many who were tested showing that they removed healthy sodium that influences potassium and created more problems. Most Americans eat too much salt but once again, it depends on your biochemical type.

This is the latest information we health professionals are being brought up to date from The Institute of Medicine: "Despite public health efforts over the past several decades to encourage people in the United States to consume less sodium, adults still consume an average of 3,400 mg/day, well above the current federal guideline of 2,300 mg or less daily. Evidence has shown that reducing sodium intake reduces blood pressure and the risk of cardiovascular disease and stroke. Some recent research, however, suggests that sodium intakes that are low may also increase health risks—particularly in certain groups." A sodium blood test is part of the normal blood tests doctors can test for to make sure you are not salting your food into an unhealthy range.

There are myths about blood pressure and they start from high blood pressure is no big deal, and everyone has high blood pressure once in a while. Or you may have heard or read that there is nothing you can do about high blood pressure - which is wrong. We always have choice, and weight control is one of the biggest. Having mentioned those myths, I do want to make sure you understand that if your blood pressure remains on the high side you must have some direction on how to treat it.

Biochemical Types Two and Three are the ones most susceptible to hypertension. The reasons are clear—both body types go for strong-flavored, spicy foods with high sodium content. In addition, these types are drawn to fatty proteins. I have discovered that when the proper biochemical diet is followed and enzyme deficiencies are replaced, the patient is once again in control of his own blood pressure. By the way, these types tend to hold their emotions inside and do not share with others.

CHILDHOOD ABDOMINAL PAIN LINKED TO ADULT ANXIETY

Before we go further into the body and anxiety I want to make you aware of the most recent problems our children are facing. It is called functional abdominal pain (FAP). Two studies presented at the Anxiety Disorders Association of America 32nd Annual Conference suggest that treating anxiety reduces both gastrointestinal and psychiatric symptoms. The studies show that the early diagnosis and treatment of pediatric anxiety can have a significant impact on the adult brain-gut connection.

"It's a bidirectional relationship. If you have anxiety and depression, you're more likely to have FAP; if you have FAP, you're more likely to have depression," said John Campo, MD, a pediatric psychiatrist who moderated the session. His previous research showed that 80 percent of pediatric FAP patients have current anxiety, 43 percent have current depressive disorder, and 29 percent have current major depressive disorder. His study involved children from 6.5 years through nine years old.

New work by Lynn Walker, a PhD holder from the Vanderbilt University School of Medicine in Nashville, Tennessee, has shown that children eight to 15 years of age whose abdominal pain persists to age 21 are five times more likely to have an anxiety disorder in adulthood. It continues to urge that those with pain that has resolved by 21 years are twice as likely to have an anxiety disorder. Dr. Walker's study involved 754 children, eight to 15 years of age with FAP and no identifiable organic disease.

Nine years after enrollment, 379 patients (average age, 21 years) were contacted and re-interviewed about their abdominal pain, other pain, and psychiatric symptoms. In the high-pain dysfunctional group, 60 percent of patients still had persistent abdominal pain. More than 45 percent of patients in the high-pain dysfunctional group met the criteria for a current anxiety disorder.

"The majority of those with a lifetime anxiety disorder often had an onset prior to their FAP evaluation," she said, adding that almost one in five patients in the high-pain dysfunctional group reported that they had lost a job because of illness. She commented, "Poor outcomes were driven by anxiety-related processes, including threat appraisal, fear, and avoidance."

PSYCHONEUROIMMUNOLOGY

It is difficult to fathom how emotions can trigger illness. George Solomon, MD, professor of psychiatry at UCLA and adjunct professor of psychiatry at the University of California at San Francisco, has demonstrated that emotional stress can affect the immune system. Dr. Solomon is known as the "father of psychoneuroimmunology." This new science is now taught at universities. Psychoneuroimmunology is a field of medicine, which joins immunology and neurology. It focuses on the relationship of stress upon the HPA axis (hypothalamus, adrenal, and pituitary). This lengthy word means the study of the effect of emotions on the immune system as a result of stress, can lead to a multitude of diseases and disorders. More evidence arises every year to support this discipline.

After the decision has been made to create changes in lifestyle, the body responds within a 21-day period. If you stop smoking or overeating or taking a health care product it paves the way for the healing process to begin. During the second 21-day period, the body begins to balance, adjust to, or accept the changes. In the third 21-day period, the body undergoes transformation. This gives the mind an adequate length of time to adjust to the change and continue healing in a positive and beneficial manner. These 21-day segments of response to change and therapy are an established regimen among health care practitioners. Although we may feel better immediately when we begin a new program, there is a period of adjustment while our bodies seek their comfort zone. Response is heightened in the second period. In the third, the condition or problem that prompted us to take action has definitely improved for the better. This is why my answer to the question about how long we need to be on a program like enzyme therapy is, "Anywhere from six to nine weeks."

If my book has inspired any of my readers to take supplemental plant-based enzymes, they may have to adjust the number of capsules taken with meals during the first 21 days. Your goal may be to improve your digestion, or to take a formulation that feeds and fortifies your hormones. For example, a client who is on a set formulation calls to say that the results first experienced have now changed. I will make the appropriate adjustment of the number of capsules taken, to meet this new need. This is a very normal scenario, and one that is frequently experienced. If you have ever tried to stop smoking or eating chocolate, you find the first three to seven days the most difficult. The remainder of the time finds the need or desire much alleviated. This is how and why I advise clients to make periodic adjustments.

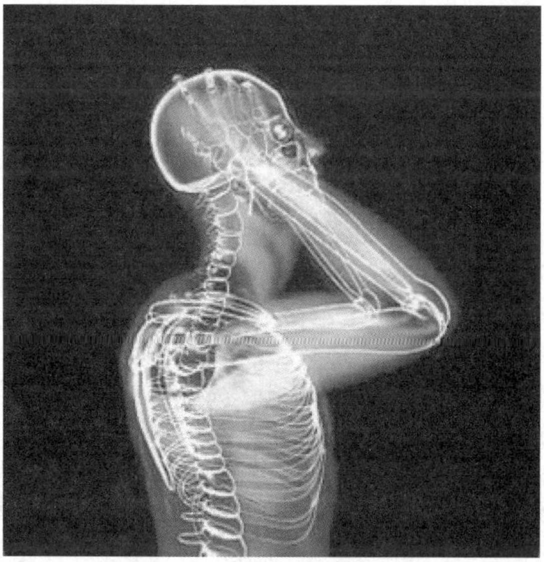

Another way to use the science of psychoneuroimmunology is to interview cancer patients or those with other catastrophic diseases. You will be surprised to find that most of them suffered some form of trauma two or more years before the onset of their illnesses. This trauma could be the death of a loved one or surviving a serious automobile accident or any other devastating experience. Some people have actually gotten so involved in their own illness they have precipitated a depressive effect onto the immune system.

I recently lost a friend, Dr. Candace Pert, who wrote a book I have referred many to throughout the years, *Molecules of Emotion*. Candace spent the last 30 years of her life devoted to the message that when we have a negative thought or feeling, it is registered throughout our bodies in moments. When asked what she felt was first as in the chicken and egg—the body or the mind—she always answered, "The bodymind . . . " they are not separate.

Dr. Bernard Siegel has stated on his tapes *Life, Hope and Healing* (Nightingale Conant) that he believes that surviving cancer has as much to do with our mental attitude as it does with the extent of our disease. I definitely agree with both him and Candace . . . My own personal experience with cancer proved this to me beyond all doubt. When I finally realized this, I no longer had to blame myself. Rather, I learned my lessons from it and went on to make the positive changes I needed to remain alive, healthy, and happy.

TESTIMONIALS

> *"Dr. DicQie I want to thank you from the bottom of my heart for the positive difference you have made in our family's life. I say family because when one of us is down it affects all of us in ways I could not before this imagine. When my daughter first started complaining about not feeling well enough to go to school, I simply put it down as being a teenager. After a time, her complaints turned into unbelievable headaches and slight rise of temperature. We began the test of time by going from doctor to doctor. Only thing that changed were their specialties. Many of the tests were evasive and always followed with some medication. The first few days we would begin to have hope but only to have it turn out sometimes worse than before we went. Thank God I heard about you from another mother who was going through something similar with her son and stomach aches. You educated us in nutrition, especially sugar, and what it does to the brain. The enzymes made such a difference and helped so very much. Your protocol, understanding, and the correct choices for all of use gave us back our joy. Know that we love you." - N. Lewis - Oregon*

"My mother complained of extreme gall bladder pain and inflammation and had a referral to visit with a surgeon to have it removed. After only being on your digestive enzymes and gastrointestinal soothing formula with each meal for a week, her pain was gone and the surgeon decided that surgery was not necessary. She was able to avoid losing a vital organ and the recovery time associated with surgery. And she felt so good, she told my Aunt who was taking two capsules of the highest strength prescription proton pump daily for extreme acid reflux. After taking digestive enzymes with each meal for one week, she no longer needs her medication at all!" - J. Buchman - Pearland, TX

"Before I placed my first order, I received a few samples and distributed the samples to my necessary patients. They really liked your digestive enzymes. An 82-year-old lady suffering with indigestion and lower abdominal pain and a 38-year-old lady with chronic discomfort in lower abdomen—these two ladies loved your products. Therefore, I decided to include digestive enzymes with every nutritional protocol in my clinic. Personally I think that your digestive enzyme is super-duper product." - S. Ahm, DC - Dallas. TX

Chapter 9

Attack the Bad Guys!

DOES YOUR IMMUNE SYSTEM REALLY NEED TO BE BALANCED OR REBUILT?

ABSOLUTELY! DO YOU KNOW WHY?

There are dozens of bad guys attacking the very system designed to do its own attacking. The main task of the immune system is to destroy toxins and other foreign invaders that take an enormous toll on the body. If you are old enough to read this book, your immune system is old enough to need continuous attention.

Of course, the first thing we all need to do is minimize our intake of bad guys. This means avoiding food and water containing agricultural chemicals, as well as limiting sugar, which stresses our pancreas, kidneys, and liver. In addition, we should cut back on simple carbohydrates that begin depressing the immune system less than an hour after we eat them.

We need to think twice about eating hormone-fed and injected meat, due to all the poisons that existed in the animal before it was killed. Purchasing grass-fed beef and organic poultry is a must. Three more items that we cannot omit from our list are stress reduction, regular exercise, and positive thinking all the time. I must admit that after writing this paragraph, I was tempted to become depressed too.

Yet, if we desire total health, none of these are exaggerations. If we work hard at the prevention process and eat a nutritional diet, our bodies will produce several million immune cells daily and earn the title "healthy." Unfortunately, the majority of us have many reasons for not practicing prevention. The result is that we put our immune systems on red alert.

OUR IMMUNE SYSTEM—WHERE IS IT LOCATED?

When we talk about the immune system, can we picture where it is in the body? There are 11 systems that run the body, and we know where most of them reside. When we think of the Cardiovascular System we picture the heart and its arteries. Urinary System makes us visualize the kidneys and bladder. Endocrine System—we may think of the thyroid, adrenal for two major ones.

Our pancreas is part of two systems (endocrine and digestive). Muscular System involves our three types of muscle groups. Nervous System consists of the brain, spinal cord, second brain and sensory organs that carry messages throughout the body. Reproductive System is made of our sex organs. Respiratory System is one that we immediately think of as our lungs. Skeletal System is another easy

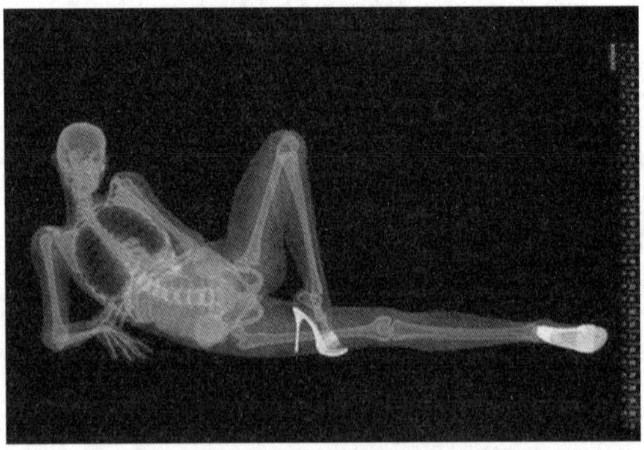

one and we picture our bones. Skin is a system for itself and the largest organ of the body. The two systems left are the Digestive and our Lymphatic (Immune) Systems.

All the systems work together to keep us alive, but the one system that helps control each of the other systems is our Digestive System. One cannot work without the others keeping it in balance (homeostasis). However, the Digestive System contains over 80 percent of the Immune System and the second brain. I hope this helps you understand why certain foods can disrupt our immune system.

AS IMPORTANT AS "BALANCE OF ALL THINGS" IS TO NATURE, SO IS THE HEALTH TO THE HUMAN BODY

The common denominator among my clients with serious conditions related to a depressed immune system is an inability to digest food properly. Some of the most common of these disorders are Epstein-Barr virus, Chronic Fatigue Syndrome, Systemic Candidiasis, and HIV infection. When poor digestion occurs, the food we eat is not broken down into the basic building blocks needed to rebuild cells and generate energy for metabolism. This brings on two big negatives: cell starvation and the release of partially digested food particles into the bloodstream.

Starved cells cause malnourished tissue that puts the brakes on important chemical processes. This results in less excretion of the toxins out of the cells. If that is the case, then fewer nutrients are introduced into the cells. There is less energy production for all cells, including those of the immune system. This reduces the number of white blood cells that are critical for fighting infection. Overall cell weakness starves the body of fuel and oxygen. A very high percentage of the population suffers from incomplete digestion, but they have yet to develop serious immune system disorders.

When the body releases partially digested food remnants into the system, it creates at least three major pathological problems:

(1) These remnants become irritants, causing inflammation of the mucosal wall of the intestines that in return releases powerful and damaging chemicals. These chemicals injure the intestinal wall enough to increase its permeability. The foreign proteins in the undigested food can leak directly into the lymphatic channels of the intestinal wall and gain access to the body's entire circulation system. Here they are considered foreign objects, so the defense mechanism mobilizes an attack by the fighter cells of the immune system. Ultimately, the battle-weary soldiers begin to run out of fuel and fail to reproduce sufficient numbers of white cells.

(2) Food remnants also provide fuel for the overgrowth of fermentative fungal organisms such as Candida Albicans and other parasites that further drain the immune system.

(3) The general inflammation brought by these wandering particles causes metabolic reactions that consume large amounts of oxygen. This produces free radicals that damage cell membranes.

Other, more complex damage occurs as well, but the medical terms and explanations are more intimidating and confusing. It is sufficient to say that the combined effects of poor digestion and errant food remnants clearly work together. They bring about a vicious sequence of events that leads to an obvious and progressive weakening of the immune system.

I have had many clients in my office over the years with Candida overgrowth and other yeast infections. Even after reading several books on the subject and trying extreme diets, each one of them remains extremely fatigued. They have a desperate look about them. By the time they get to me they have tried so many things and have spent enormous amounts of money. These clients challenge me to help them.

Candidiasis is one of the many fungal forms known to the human body that can become imbalanced. I have met with several Candidiasis support groups and it is amazing to see how much freedom they have gained simply by understanding the real nature of the illness. Candida is natural to the body and only becomes candidiasis (overgrowth) when the immune system is not functioning efficiently. Fatigue and depression are two of the most significant symptoms. Good diet alone cannot control these symptoms. We must evaluate the individual body's inability to break down foods that compromise their immune system.

I do not put anyone on an extreme diet or regimen. I suggest they learn about their biochemical types and which foods sustain them. Many people ask me questions about diet. Some ask specifically why others can easily eat mushrooms, but they cannot. It is not because mushroom is a fungus; rather it is the inability to break down the mushroom, an important factor. The answer can usually be found in one's genes or enzyme potential. A big part of my practice involves working with people who have fungal problems. We must always consider individual Biochemical type and how the same food can affect a dozen different people with 12 different reactions. The only food that seems to cause havoc for everyone if eaten in excess is sugar. Within weeks after treatment began, dramatic changes took place in the lives of these clients. I observed a big improvement. Later in this chapter, I will discuss Candida overgrowth in more detail.

RELIEF FOR EAR INFECTIONS

Ear infections are very common among teenagers and younger children. These are the ages when children tend to eat a great deal of sugar and other junk food. This only worsens their condition. The amount of mucus in their systems increases due to a poor selection of foods. The immune system is depressed. When I complete a Live Cell Analysis on them, they all have fungal forms in common. I suggest they take high dosages of protease between meals to boost the immune system. I encourage all of them to pay close attention to how much sugar and other junk food they are eating. A multiple enzyme product will counteract their poor digestion if taken at meal times. These multiple enzymes must be taken with snacks as well. Children love to snack after school or while watching TV. Parents are responsible for keeping the enzymes handy if they want to prevent sluggish immune systems in their children. Doctors involved in enzyme therapy begin babies on enzymes as soon as they are home from the hospital. They use only pharmaceutical-grade plant enzymes without fillers.

BRUISING: A SIGN OF DEFICIENCY

Normal bruising is not a concern if it happens from bumping into something or perhaps a fall. These bruises fade within a normal time period. There are many people who bruise quite easily, especially as they age. Those bruises tend to linger a long while before they fade. As we age, our ability to make digestive enzymes is lessened, and this leads to a needy and deficient state of health. In preventive medicine, bruising is always a sign of someone lacking nutrients and at least a slightly depressed immune system. If you fall into this category, I suggest you try the natural digestive enzymes for support in delivering natural nutrients.

We can take vitamins and minerals in whole food or synthetic form. This does not mean they are always delivered to our cells. I recommend you do some research of your own, and look at the studies showing most people to be nutrient deficient. Many eat the best quality foods and take what they regard as good vitamin supplements. Yet they still bruise easily or catch cold frequently. Taking vitamins and minerals does not necessarily mean that the nutrient deficiency will be relieved immediately. If it's not the right balance of nutrients for your biochemical type (genetic needs), you won't have the expected results.

Find out what caused the problem. Quite likely it will be a case of toxicity in the system. We do not realize that synthetic vitamins (those that are measured in milligrams as Vitamin C 1000 mg) can be part of our toxicity. We can cause a toxic reaction by taking improper nutrients. A toxic body is a deficient body. A man-made vitamin (in a lab) outside of a food is a reflection of itself. In other words, it is like you are looking into a mirror and you see yourself, but out of the two of you, only one is real and the other a reflection. When the body needs a nutrient it will use an enzyme to have it delivered.

The metabolic enzyme your body makes can only deliver a part of the synthetic version and the rest results in a toxin to be taken from the system. Hence expensive vitamins in the urine! For instance, we can only absorb a set amount of nutrients into the cell in a period of time. Example is zinc we only can absorb anywhere from 3 to 5 mg of zinc dependent on our size in 24 hours. A doctor friend called to tell me he found a zinc product that is 85 mg. I had to caution him that his body would have the added toxicity of getting rid of the synthetic 80 mg.

Highly toxic conditions manifest in various ways. It is best to treat toxicity and deficiency at the same time. Before we knew about the miraculous properties of supplemental plant-based enzymes, it was nearly impossible to do so. Now we can assist digestion by cutting back on the cause of the toxic state. It is now possible to assist digestion and the enzymes break loose the nutrients, which they deliver directly to our cell. We can cleanse and fortify the liver and blood along with feeding and reinforcing the glandular and nervous systems. Within a short period of time, the bruises will fade and will not return. What makes it so rewarding for me is that my clients can see and feel the difference in their health. At the end of this chapter you will find more information on enzyme dosages.

Overweight people have a continual battle to fight between the excess body fat they carry and their immune systems. The weaker their immune systems, the more they are subject to colds, flu, serious infections, viruses, heart disease, diabetes, and degenerative disorders. What is worse, when the immune system is depressed, the body is much more prone to weight gain. This causes an emotionally painful, self-perpetuating cycle. Only one of the four biochemical types, Type Three, can carry extra pounds and not suffer fatigue or a depressed immune system. However, if high blood pressure, constipation, or insomnia develops, the Type Three will also contract trouble with the immune system. The final result is that they, too, will be as vulnerable as the other three-biochemical types.

THE COMMON COLD SHOULD NOT BE COMMON

The common cold is an acute and highly contagious virus infection of the upper respiratory tract. At least 20 identifiable viruses have been found to cause colds, and they attack anyone with weakened resistance. It has been my experience that almost all of my clients who take enzymes consistently no longer have the colds that plagued them many times throughout the year.

How is this possible? I believe it is because they are finally digesting their food completely, eliminating undigested food particles out of their systems! Those food particles create distress and harbor bacteria that depress our immune systems. Types One and Two tend to be mucus makers because of poor digestion. If you are looking for total health, it is so important for you to educate yourself about all causes of poor health. Be certain you know the facts about the sugars, the nutrient robbers, and mucus makers. If this is not enough to convince you, go back and reread the sections that deal with sugar intolerance.

SAY GOODBYE TO CANDIDIASIS

Candida, a yeast-like fungus, is one of the many fungal forms that can create problems in the human body (known as Candidiasis.) There are 13 different fungi that can be detected using Live Blood Analysis. They all share the ability to cause fatigue and many other debilitating conditions. I will not spend much time here on the problem of Candida. Hundreds of books and diets on the subject are on the market. Remember, these diets only work while you are closely following them. The stress suffered from following the diet is almost as great as the Candida.

To keep it very simple, the fungal forms are proteins. When we take protease between meals to consume the excess radical protein, we have done away with the cause of the Candida. The formulation I recommend is at least 600,000 units of protease activity three to five times a day. In the practice of enzyme nutrition, health professionals sometime give over 3 million units of protease in one day.

I suggest the food plan corresponding to your biochemical type. In addition, you need the proper enzymes for support of the endocrine system along with the miracle-working protease to digest the spores of the fungal forms.

I believe it is important for you to have more information on the part played by the microorganisms (probiotics), which live in our intestines. They are critical to our good health. We carry more than four hundred species of indigenous bacteria that are constant companions to our intestinal tracts. Our health is maintained by keeping them in balance, so that no one organism becomes dominant among this flora. Normally, the resident bacteria preserve this balance. We are subject to both internal and external stresses that can interrupt the balance. If the balance is tipped and an overgrowth of yeast organisms occurs, they overwhelm the normal bacteria in the colon.

The most common of these overgrowths is Candida Albicans.

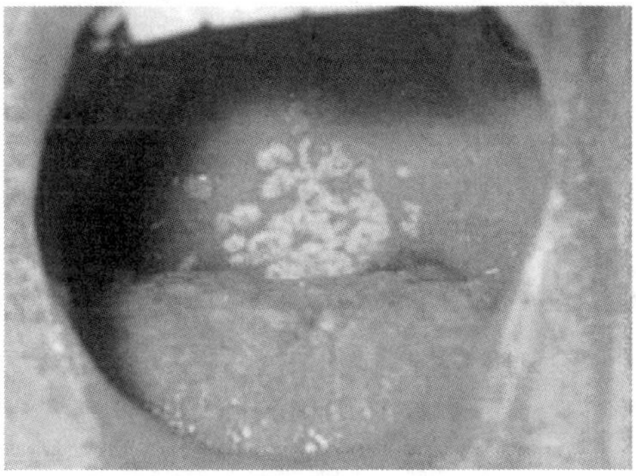

Candida is only a problem if the overgrowth occurs. A certain amount of this fungus is normal and healthy in the human body. This is also why we cannot rid it totally from the body system. What does this overgrowth look like and how does it make us feel? Symptoms will vary. Candidiasis is found in 70 percent of our population. Sometimes thrush develops in the mouth. Women often get vaginal yeast infections.

Three systems are most profoundly affected by Candida: the gastrointestinal, urinary, and respiratory tracts. An imbalance in the gastrointestinal tract will cause bloating, poor absorption of vitamins and minerals, food allergies, sensitivity, nausea, and diarrhea. Imbalances in the urinary tract produce frequent urination, pain, burning, swelling, and a strong odor. The respiratory tract becomes susceptible to bronchitis, chronic sinusitis, or postnasal drip.

Bloating and inability to tolerate various vitamins or nutrients are the most common of the Candida symptoms. Candida can directly cause a high incidence of food intolerance. Many more women have Candida because of birth control pills. Those who take frequent or massive dosages of antibiotics, such as tetracycline, are very much prone to Candida because the medication destroys the natural balance of healthy bacteria in the intestines. If you eat too much sugar or simple carbohydrates, you are more susceptible. Women who douche too often will destroy the balance of healthy bacteria in the vagina.

Fungal infections can range in severity from superficial to life threatening. For example, fungal infections affecting only the top layers of the skin are readily treatable and have a relatively limited impact on quality of life. However, if a fungal infection enters systemic circulation, consequences can be deadly.

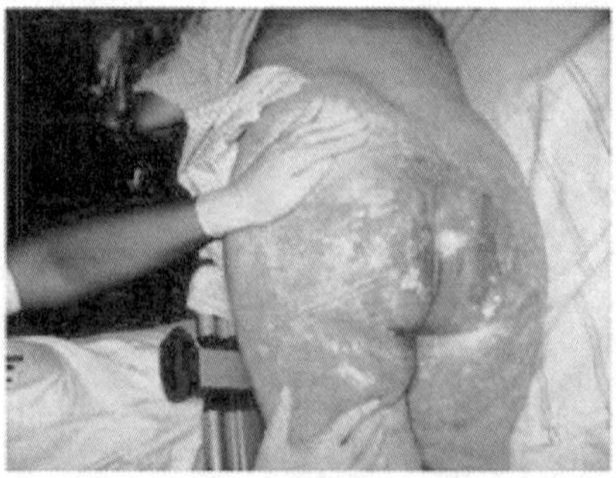

Protease is the best of the enzyme types for treatment of Candida. Candida or fungal is called unicellular—meaning it is a single cell. Protease rids our systems of the excessive growth of any of the fungal forms without side effects. As with most illnesses and other health problems, the best treatment for Candida is to create a healthy internal environment. Many different products are on the market for our use. The needs for bactocilli and bifidus products are common knowledge to anyone who has ever been formally diagnosed with Candida. However, I believe that many of the new bacteria such as *L. Plantarum* and *L. Salvarius* are superior. Different bacteria can be used together to create balance. *L. Plantarum* has over 200 billion organisms with a growth rate that doubles in less than five minutes. That is a big improvement over the acidophilus we used in the past. Bacteria are preventative and precautionary measures for balancing the system. I favor their use because in the right combination, they balance the pH and the bacteria of the small and large intestines as well. Remember, your small and large intestines are the last places good digestion can occur, so it is critical that proper balance is maintained in them. If not, fungal forms will take over.

Candida albicans does not have a long history. Research shows it came on the scene about the same time we started to eat too much sugar. Another event that contributed to its growth was the advent of widespread use of antibiotics, beginning in the 1940s and 1950s. Those who have the worst symptoms and the most acute emotional depression are the ones who have Candida and hypoglycemia simultaneously.

To sum up, the best approach for prevention is to add enzyme supplements to the daily diet, and eliminate sugar. Please be aware of your sugar intake. If you will not cut back on sugar, at least add the enzymes. Some of the food will be digested, some of the nutrients will be delivered, and some of the mess will get cleaned up. To get rid of the invaders, the use of protease between meals will start the correction process.

Precautionary measures make a great deal of sense to me. When clients come in for a consultation, I do not ask for radical changes. I make suggestions and give choices. However, the bottom line on sugar is...it's out! An absolute NO to fructose, sugar, and sugar substitutes which have even more side effects. This does not mean that a piece of raw fruit can't be good for you, but avoid fruit juices because of the excessive sugar content. It is really quite simple. Read the labels on food products when you are grocery shopping. Choose only those items that are not high in sugar or simple carbohydrates. The benefits you will feel are worth the effort.

It is very difficult for Americans to overcome their sweet tooth. I feel it would be far easier to give up the sweets and start to rebuild our systems, rather than suffer the aches, pains, and swelling that come with a strong sugar habit. I have found that when we take doses of carbohydrate-splitting and protease enzymes together, the swelling and inflammation in the body begins to dissipate right away. The client feels an almost immediate difference.

This takes place after using these miraculous supplemental plant-based enzymes. We do know that carbohydrate-splitting enzymes with meals and proteases in large doses are perfect for those who suffer from Candida overgrowth and chronic fatigue syndrome. However, I would never formulate a regimen with just one (carbo-splitting enzyme) called amylase, because I know the importance of the enzymes' working together. Some formulas have high amylase and cellulose, but it is not reaching the spore.

CASE HISTORY

One of my women clients, a very successful surgical nurse, suffered from candidiasis. After going through the standard medications she was prescribed for it, she was still very lethargic. She felt she had lost her zest for living. She became so exhausted she had to give up her practice. Her skin broke out, and she gained a lot of weight. When she came to my office, I explained how I look at the body's natural processes.

From that moment, I told her we would not fight against her illness; we would simply create an environment where the invaders could no longer live. This, of course, comes through the use of supplemental enzymes. She began with high dosages of protease between meals, three to five times per day. Along with this, she took the multi-digestive enzymes for more efficient digestion. This client learned that she could no longer afford to leave undigested food particles in her system. I also gave her herbs mixed with the enzymes. These can be taken in very small amounts, because the enzymes will deliver them to the cells.

The two of them make a very successful health-care team. We paid close attention to her endocrine and immune systems. Within a month, she was back to work. In six weeks, she was completely up to speed. Today, she is still doing beautifully. We have remained in contact through the years. I can call on her for support for those who are desperate and feel there is no way out of the traps they have laid for themselves. It gives us a great sense of freedom to realize we can take control of our health, and we can restore balance to the entire body.

UNHEALTHY CONDITIONS IN THE INTESTINAL TRACT ARE ANY PARASITE'S DREAM

Unhealthy and imbalanced intestinal tract is the ideal environment for parasites. There are at least 134 varieties of parasites that can thrive in the human body. Americans are infested with parasites due to our polluted water system, junk foods, too many cooked foods, and a lack of raw fruits and vegetables in our diets. Researchers in the health care field estimate there are 200 million people in this country who are infested with intestinal parasites. Once they enter the intestinal tract, parasites have easy access to all parts of the body. They can cause a number of diseases.

Parasites, viruses, fungal forms, and bacteria are protein in composition. Because these offenders are proteins, the enzyme protease works wonders in their destruction. Without any side effects, we can fend off these attackers of our immune system. Here is an example of how protease works. We all know that ear infections are a common affliction in both children and adults. The virus causing the infection has a protein coating that protects the spore, the actual culprit. Protease digests the coating and exposes the spore to the white blood cells waiting to pounce upon it! I think that is an absolute miracle of nature, and in particular the design of the human body.

Parasites occur naturally in the body. They are everywhere. We get them from human contact. We can pick them up from walking barefooted or in the food we eat. However, when parasites are out of control and become toxic, we have health problems. This is what happens in the case of the Candida fungus. Its presence in the intestine is normal until overgrowth occurs through autointoxication. Then it develops into candidiasis, which is abnormal. Those familiar with the practice of colon cleansing know there is a specific place in the colon known as the region of parasites. In order to remove the parasites, it is essential to embark upon an effective elimination program. Parasites can be destroyed harmlessly and without side effects of drugs. Ingesting protease enzymes safely accomplishes this. They are nontoxic and natural. Great diligence is required on the part of the client. You must take the capsules with consistency and a real dedication to your cleansing program. When you do, the rewards are enormous.

A few years ago, scientists did not recognize phytochemicals. Yet today they are the new frontier in cancer-prevention research. The word is derived from the Greek, meaning, "plant." Newsweek magazine dedicated five pages to an article titled "Beyond Vitamins" in its April 25, 1994 issue. It stated that raw vegetables and fruit such as tomatoes, apricots, and broccoli contain thousands of phytochemicals.

These substances work by waking up enzymes inside cells and detoxifying cancer-causing chemicals. This article came out just after The New England Journal of Medicine delivered a pessimistic message about those vitamins known as antioxidants. The holistic health community's long-awaited verdict in the "great vitamin debate" did not give the vitamin industry the break it wanted. Nonetheless, scientists reported information on a "magic pill," one that would go beyond vitamins.

A compound called sulforaphane, derived from broccoli, cauliflower, brussels sprouts, turnips, and kale was discovered that kept laboratory animals free of cancer. Early in the 1990s, research with cells in a lab dish led biochemists to suspect that sulforaphane works its magic by boosting the activity of phase two enzymes. These enzymes detoxify carcinogens by hooking them up to molecules and moving them out of the cells where they are rendered harmless. Phytochemicals in strawberries, grapes, and raspberries also neutralize carcinogens before they can invade DNA. It is called elegiac acid.

Even if these early preventatives fail, there is yet another pre-cancer instance where phytochemicals can intervene. In 1993, German researchers announced that they had isolated a chemical in soybeans that prevents the attack of cancer cells in the bloodstream. This chemical is a growth inhibitor of cancer. Supplemental plant-based enzymes have the same capabilities as these compounds like sulforaphane or the phytochemicals. Their action in the stomach assists the digestion and breakdown of the foods. Ingested on an empty stomach, they can clean up the blood, improve circulation, and blood rheology. Enzyme action is very much like cellular musical chairs.

These compounds race to sites on the cell where cancer-causing hormones, including improper estrogen, attach themselves. When the music stops, the enzymes keep the hormones from sitting on the cell's surface. The protease enzymes do even a greater job since they can break down the surface or coating of the cancer cell and expose it to the host to immune system. After the information came out about the research on phytochemicals, several new products appeared on the shelves at health food stores. These products contained freeze-dried vegetables. Claims were made that salads or juices could be ingested in capsule form. In truth, we have known about research and information concerning supplemental plant based enzymes for over seventy years. When these products are touted as new ones, it really means they are brand new only to the writer of the article.

CARDIOVASCULAR DISEASE

Cardiovascular disease is not limited to the elderly; age has nothing to do with it. Enzyme therapy is used successfully to treat diseases of the arteries and veins. In their book, *Enzymes: The Fountain of Life*, Drs. Lopez, Williams, and Miehlke offer evidence for this. Studies continue to a great extent in Europe, and some in the United States, supporting the use of enzymes. To quote Dr. Inderst in a lecture from September 12, 1990: "Enzyme Therapy is a proven treatment and method for disease relating to blood vessels. It diminishes the swelling, activates the system, and stimulates cells such as macrophages (white blood cells) without the long-term side effects of drug therapy."

Besides being the number one killer disease in America, heart or cardiovascular disease is one of the leading causes of disability. How can this happen? To best understand this complex and critically important part of the body, let us discuss the cardiovascular system. The primary focus of this system is to move blood throughout the body. It is made up of the heart, blood vessels, and lymph vessels.

The circulatory system transports oxygen, nutrients, immune system secretions, hormones, and chemicals necessary for normal function and activity of the organs. It also carries away waste products and carbon dioxide. This miraculous system equalizes body temperature and helps to maintain normal water and electrolyte balance (salt and potassium).

An adult has an average of six quarts of blood in his body. The circulatory system carries this entire quantity through one complete circuit of the body every minute. In the course of 24 hours, 7,200 quarts of blood pass through the heart. Very small vessels, known as capillaries, are so tiny the blood cells must enter them single file. The rate of blood flow through the vessels depends on several factors. These are: force of the heartbeat, rate of the heartbeat, control of the quantity of blood that enters the heart chambers, and finally, the capillaries.

The blood then returns to the heart by flowing through the veins, and the process begins again. The circulation of the blood is extremely important. As it passes through the arteries and veins in the heart, neck, head, brain, and digestive organs, it delivers and picks up carbohydrates, proteins, fats, and chemicals. When blood enters and exits the liver, it brings glucose and glycogen and removes toxins. In the kidneys, it cleanses. In the lymphatic glands, it delivers nutrients. And in organs like the spleen, tonsils, and thymus, it supports the immune system.

The organs and systems of the body vary greatly in the quantity of blood they require at different times. For instance, the brain needs a great deal of blood all the time. Muscles demand blood sporadically. Many things depend on physical exertion, which increases the blood flow to the muscles. Hot weather increases the flow of blood to cool the body. Whenever we eat a meal, extra blood is required by the stomach to help digest and absorb the food.

The nervous system controls all this activity. Without this vital control, none of the various needs for blood could be maintained. If the nervous system was not doing its job, the quantity of blood in the brain would change if you shift the position of your body even slightly. There are two nerves that control blood supply. One is located in the heart; the other one is in the neck. These two nerves are perfectly synchronized.

They register any changes in the blood pressure and cause the nervous system to change the rate of heartbeat and the size of the blood vessels to always maintain correct blood pressure. Perhaps now you understand the importance of the circulatory system and how our very life depends on its precision work. It is yet another of the marvels and miracles of our bodies.

Lipase enzymes are the major enzymes used for the breakdown of fats and cholesterol and also for lipid regulation. Recently, a cardiologist whom I know admitted that if the public understood the capabilities of lipase, there would no longer be a need for him to continue his medical practice. I thought that was quite a statement! Obviously this is overstated since hereditary heart diseases would always create a need for cardiologists.

Lipase is used with other plant-based enzymes to assist with proper digestion. This feeds and cleanses the life-giving blood in the body. Every red cell has an outer lipid lining. Enzymatic action runs the life force in our bodies—every thought, every breath. Our entire being is enzyme-dependent.

Do I believe enzymes are important? What do you think, since they assist in the breakdown of food, delivery of nutrients, and fortification of the blood? If used correctly, are they the very life source for our kidneys, liver, brain, and lungs? I answer with an absolute yes to all these questions! My observation of those with heart problems suggests that elimination of sugars and simple carbohydrates from the diet is an excellent starting point.

Frequent urination is a difficulty people with heart conditions face. This is because their doctors have prescribed diuretics to help control hypertension and a disturbed heart rhythm. However, when the client gets rid of excess sugar consumption, the blood sugar level begins to stabilize. Only then can the body start to eliminate toxins naturally. The medications being taken are reduced to a lower dosage.

Heart disease is an area of great interest to me because my mother and my sister suffered from it. When I was with my mother, I noticed that control of her diet has a direct effect on her heart rhythm and how often she urinates. Blood vessels are just as biologically active as the liver, kidneys, or any other vital organ. The blood vessels depend on enzymes. When the blood vessels are clogged with fats the effectiveness of the enzymes is reduced. The blood vessels can become constricted. How can someone who is interested in prevention deal with this?

Keep your enzymes working all the time! Everything that happens in the body does so because of these miraculous substances. As we become more stressed or ill, our immune system suffers and the power of the enzymes is seriously undermined as well. It makes so much sense to take supplemental digestive enzyme in order to feed and fortify the body. This takes pressure off the digestive system, allowing it to function more efficiently. Plant-based supplemental enzymes keep our blood healthy, and helps keep our systems in balance.

ARTHRITIS

In 2010, it was estimated that 50 million Americans suffer with diagnosed Arthritis. Arthritis treatment costs the nation $150 billion every year. Incidence of arthritis is expected to skyrocket as baby boomers begin to turn 50. By the year 2020, more than 60 million people will have some form of arthritis, states Dr. Charles Helmick of the Centers for Disease Control and Prevention. Women are especially susceptible. One in five women has arthritis compared to only 12 percent of men. Medical terminology uses the suffix "-itis" to describe disorders involving inflammation. A partial list of these includes arthritis, pancreatitis, dermatitis, and prostatitis.

Rheumatoid arthritis is systemic, meaning it is present throughout the body and involves the connective tissue. Degenerative lesions may be found in the collagen (a fibrous protein in connective tissue, bone, and cartilage) of the lungs, heart, blood vessels, and pleura. Those who suffer from the rheumatoid variety often appear to be undernourished and chronically ill because of the inflammation of blood-forming organs. Most common is the arthritis that attacks the joints. Osteoarthritis is located in the musculoskeletal system (muscle and skeleton). Arthritis is one of the most difficult conditions to treat.

The drugs used for treatment stop the body from making prostaglandins. While prostaglandins are responsible for the swelling of the joints, they also protect the stomach from acids and other digestive juices necessary to dissolve food. As a result, about 15 percent of all arthritic people have ulcers. The goal for medical technology is to develop a drug that reduces swelling without disturbing the stomach. Many of the other treatments have harmful side effects that lead to other diseases. No matter what the treatment or side effects are for arthritis, the one certainty is it interferes with quality of life.

The consistency of the blood changes and more white blood cells are created as a result of inflammation. This is how the body naturally reacts and attempts to protect itself. A positive response to inflammation depends on adequate protease enzymes. If the inflammation is constant or the onset of it is especially severe, an increased abundance of internal support enzymes is required. However, the quantities needed are too great for the body to produce without assistance. The body is unable to radically change its rate of enzyme production, just as it is incapable of drastically slowing it. The significance of a constant, steady supply of enzymes cannot be overemphasized.

When the body's immune (defense) system breaks down, it is because of an internal enzyme shortage. This begins a process called autoimmunity. The body begins to regard its own tissue or cell structure as a foreign invader. Our immune system begins to fight against itself. It attacks its own connective tissue, joints, skin, and blood cells.

While this battle rages, the original disorder is still taking its toll. The outcome is chronic illness. In autoimmune disorders, I see some common denominators. Most of those who suffer have problems digesting fats and protein. They tend to be either Biochemical Type Two or Three. They prefer heavily spiced, strong-flavored foods, crave sugar, and were raised on meat. Does this mean they will never eat meat or spicy food again? No, it means that these are the cravings of most arthritic people I have counseled.

Protease and lipase are the enzymes they need the most. The case histories are numerous. They are all very much the same. This is why I approach all the autoimmune disorders with the same enzyme regimen. First, I address the primary problem of poor digestion with a multiple-enzyme supplement taken with every meal. High dosages of protease are taken between meals for the antioxidant properties.

Most of these clients are constipated. I suggest the use of a bacterium-fortified enzyme with herb formulation to assist with frequent, healthy bowel movements. Without exception, all systems are very toxic. With the aid of supplemental plant-based enzymes we feed, fortify, and detoxify.

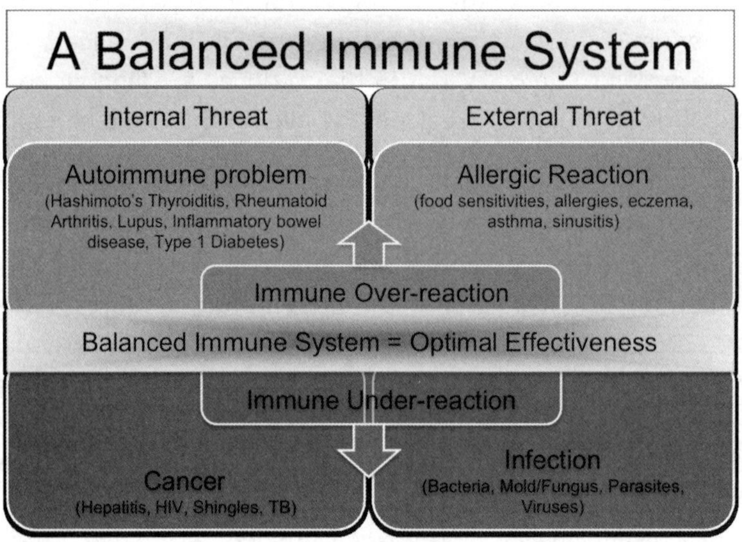

IMMUNE BOOSTERS: "THE ENZYME CONNECTION"

In thousands of my clients' case histories, enzyme supplements produced a stunning turnaround. This amazed themselves but also their families, friends, and even their doctors. I am not alone among health-care professionals who have experienced this. Many of them have shared the same information in interviews, books, or by word-of-mouth. It seems as if enzymes play two different roles in rebuilding the immune system. First, they act as an agent that counteracts the causes of the initial damage. Then, they balance the immune system itself.

This is how it works. Supplemental digestive enzymes attack the offenders themselves by reducing inflammation and neutralizing many of the toxins that injure the mucosal wall. This reduces leakage of partially digested food remnants, mostly chunks of allergenic protein, through the intestinal walls and into the bloodstream. Our powerful protein-digesting enzymes come to the rescue. When taken on an empty stomach, it escorts the protein fragments from the small intestine into the colon where they are destroyed through normal digestive procedures. This same enzyme, when no longer needed in the intestine, moves directly into the blood. There, it continues to remove toxins and other unwanted protein matter.

Supplemental plant-based enzyme supplements help strengthen the immune system by increasing the number and intensity of the fighter cells. These warrior cells are macrophages, monocytes (large, mononuclear, non-granular white blood cells with round or kidney-shaped nuclei) and T-cells (lymphocytes involved in rejecting foreign tissue, regulating cellular immunity, and controlling the production of antibodies). When the enzymes reach these immune-system cells, they increase the fluidity and permeability of the cell membranes. This makes it much easier for nutrients to enter the cells... and much easier for toxins to leave. This creates improved cellular metabolism throughout the body and an overall boost in energy level. After the vicious cycle of malnutrition, poor digestion, and cellular starvation is finally broken, your immune system is remarkably stronger.

It has been my fortune to see the changes that enzymes make in the human blood. Working with medical doctors, I have the honor to be a consultant to some of them. This gives me the opportunity to study the experiences and case histories of many clients and patients. I feel great humility when I see an enormous transformation occur in someone who has been critically ill. One gentleman, in particular, comes to mind.

CASE HISTORY

A successful oncologist surgeon called my office on a Thursday afternoon. I clearly remember the day of the week because it plays a role in this story. The surgeon asked if he could bring one of his patients in to see me. He wanted to observe the Live Blood Analysis. This is a procedure I teach to preventative practitioners that allows them to evaluate live blood samples and teach nutrition. It is used as a teaching tool, rather than a diagnostic one. A drop of blood from the finger is placed on a microscope slide.

This technique is called dark-field microscopy. The observer can detect motion in the cells, noting balances and imbalances. The patient in question had just completed his final chemo treatment. With a dangerously low white blood count, his doctors were afraid to give him any more.

The injections he received to elevate the white count did not work. His WBC (white blood count) was 580. Normally the leukocytes should read about 8,000 WBC. His was so far below normal that his physicians were concerned he might have a compromised immune system. I knew, of course, that the enzymes would elevate the WBC. However, the surgeon was desperate. He wanted to see a detectable difference almost immediately.

The doctor intended to do another blood count on Monday morning. It was late Thursday afternoon. When someone is relatively healthy, at least not suffering from terminal illness, we can see an increase in both the WBC and RBC within 10 minutes of ingesting a protease simulation. In this case, we were able to see some new white blood cells and T-cells in a matter of a few minutes. Both the doctor and I were elated.

I explained to his patient that I had no idea until that moment that we could see results so quickly after chemo. As they were leaving, I gave the man nutrition information along with all the standard enzyme formulations. By Tuesday morning, a very happy doctor had phoned me to inform me his patient's white blood count was back up to 7,800 by the previous afternoon. The last time I saw this man he was doing very well, his cancer is in remission. His hair was growing back in, and he told me he felt wonderful. This took place over 15 years ago, and he is still well and free of cancer.

DO YOU HAVE HEALTHY BLOOD?

Do you have healthy and vigorous blood? Or is it tired and weak? The answers to these questions could very well mean the difference between a healthy, energetic lifestyle and one of constant weariness and fatigue. We cannot live without that extraordinary and complex protein fluid coursing through our bodies. A miracle of modern science is our ability to use one another's blood as long as it's the same type. The blood's liquid component is called plasma. It is the primary ingredient of this life-sustaining, homogenous mixture. The plasma functions as the carrier of food, oxygen, vitamins, and minerals to cells, in exchange for waste matter. The solid matter in blood consists almost entirely of coin-shaped red cells. Remarkably elastic, they are so flexible they can extend, fold up, and squeeze through a capillary barely half their own diameter. Red cells are naturally manufactured in our bone marrow. Their principal ingredient is hemoglobin, a protein molecule programmed to combine with oxygen. Blood contains other miraculous substances as well. One is a thin, plate-shaped cell called a platelet, which is essential for clotting. If the skin is cut, for instance, and a blood leak occurs, the platelet releases a chemical that crystallizes one of the plasma's proteins. Called fibrinogen, it creates a net or a web of red cells, all hooked together into a solid plug. The larger white blood cells, considerably less numerous than the red ones, act as the body's defense team. When an invasion of bacteria, fungal forms, or parasites occurs, white blood cells multiply as they engulf and destroy these enemies.

Our blood cannot survive or function without oxygen. The manner in which blood is oxygenated is remarkable. The average adult male has a capillary system that would stretch out, end to end, to about 60,000 miles. The lungs are fraught with these minute vessels. As we take a breath, the oxygen we inhale enters the blood through the very thin walls of these capillaries. The blood carries this oxygen to all the body's tissues. Capillaries are like garden hoses inserted into the river of an artery or vein. Each one is less than one-one thousandth of an inch in diameter. More than 3 million of them thread through each square inch in the cross section of a muscle. Each capillary carries its dribble of blood swiftly. The heart patiently pumps the body's six quarts of blood through all its tissues again and again. The average pace of a complete round trip is about one minute.

The lymph system is a companion to the circulatory, or blood system. Its primary purpose is to isolate and eliminate dangerous infections. The lymphatic system circulates more or less parallel to the blood. The lymph glands, or nodes, are made up of valves and filters, and they travel more slowly because they do not have a pump as the heart does.

Blood circulation is continuous but not constant in an active body. Muscular, electrical, and chemical controls unceasingly regulate and change the pattern of flow. It acts like a sprinkler system in your front yard where different groups of sprinkler heads open and close, flooding first one area and then another. Blood can flow like a big river, causing obstacles too big or heavy to be flushed away, sometimes even reversing the current in certain channels. The entire operation is controlled by special centers in the brain. These receive information from sensory monitoring devices located at strategic points. They send signals to the heart and to thousands of arterial, venal, and capillary control stations.

Human blood, in a nutshell, performs all these life-giving functions for our bodies:

- Circulates oxygen throughout the body's network of arteries, veins, and capillaries

- Delivers nutrients to the tissues and organs
- Carries minerals, hormones, vitamins, and antibodies
- Removes waste products

Many substances vital to health are recycled through the blood. Blood helps maintain equilibrium (homeostasis) of the internal environment. It bathes the tissue with oxygen. It collects waste products. Its major regulatory duties involve the nutrition of cells, protecting against foreign invaders, and keeping the body temperature constant. The blood also facilitates the body's adaptability to changes in external conditions. These include climatic changes, stressful physical activity, new eating habits, and resistance to injury and infectious organisms.

Blood is analyzed for information leading to nutrient deficiencies and disease. Red blood cells circulate in the bloodstream for about 120 days. After that, they are trapped and broken down in the spleen, an organ responsible for storing and filtering blood. The spleen and liver can function as backup sites for red blood cell reserves in an emergency. They act as salvage yards for iron reclaimed from dead red blood cells. The total numbers of red blood cells in the body vary with age, altitude, activity, and temperature. An average, healthy individual has about 35 trillion of them. White blood cells or leukocytes are the principal component of the body's immune system. Acting as scavengers, they assist with the repair of the body.

Blood cells are generated in the bone marrow or lymph nodes. These nodes serve as defense outposts against germs that are attacking the body. White blood cells travel from site to site through the arteries, veins, and capillaries. White cells can also leave the bloodstream and filter into the lymphatic tissues if necessary to fight infection. Although these cells are produced in large quantities, they die within a few days. Vastly outnumbered by the red blood cells, the average, healthy human has only about 75 billion leukocytes in the blood.

Personal physicians order most of the blood tests performed on human beings. The blood taken from the inner bend of your elbow at your doctor's office is almost always sent to medical laboratories for testing. However, there are ways for the layperson to observe their own live blood specimen. One method is called dark-field microscopy. I remind you that this is not used for diagnostic purposes. Rather, it is a nutritional teaching tool. I use it in our research programs. It is not approved by CLIA in America and has to be used for research in labs. Through the powerful lens of the microscope, we can observe white blood cells to see if they are doing their job efficiently. This can be an excellent indicator of the performance of the autoimmune system. Imbalances detected by the dark field microscope are based on nutritional information about the client, which shows up in blood activity. Someone who has problems digesting fats could have a buildup of platelets adhering to the walls and rough surfaces of a damaged vessel. This condition indicates high cholesterol and headaches. Poorly digested protein will show up in the plasma and will cause the red blood cells to stick to each other. When the liver is toxic from alcohol consumption, prescription drugs, or lack of digestion, it shows up as fibrin material in the plasma.

When digestion is actually in progress, blood fats are easily recognized by the dark-field method. Toxicity appears as bright, shiny crystals. These are often so toxic that they will show up in color on a black and white screen. Some deficiencies look like oval or misshapen red blood cells. In the case of a nutrient deficiency, the red blood cells cannot maintain form and simply fade from view. White blood cells are easily distinguishable and give information about the immune system. One of the most commonly occurring problems is a variation in the white blood cells, or leukocytosis. These cells are present in the blood because the body is in a state of alert against the havoc caused by poorly digested food. The body sees the undigested particles as invaders and responds by calling out the white blood cells.

Dark-field microscopy was for me instrumental in proving the importance of supplemental plant-based enzyme therapy. I tend to try new products on myself as a living laboratory. After ingesting the product, if I observe a change for the good, I am then interested in further use of it. Unfortunately, many formulations do not show a positive change. In my own experience, I have discovered that too often those taking mega-doses of vitamins and minerals can create further imbalances. This can be just as much of an upset to the body's nutrients as it is when poor nutrition occurs. A practitioner can measure these imbalances using blood, urine, and saliva. Our system is overwhelmed when we take more nutritionals than we need. Ingesting enzymes are a different matter altogether. They are catalysts that make things happen in the system. In addition, they are not stored nor can they cause an imbalance because they are proteins and can work for minutes, days or weeks dependent on the need and type. If one takes a larger amount than needed at that moment, our cells to make more metabolic enzymes use them.

CONCLUSION

The primary function of the immune system is to protect the body from infection, damage, and ultimately disease. Recurrent or chronic infections occur only when the immune system is weakened by a lack of proper nutrition or by excesses of stress, pollution, radiation, toxins, and exposure to a vast array of infectious microorganisms.

In a healthy lymphatic system, the initial exposure to these offending agents' creates an allergic reaction, an inflammatory response, and then healing. However, long-term exposure without proper support to the immune system, may lead to chronic allergies, systemic inflammation, and oxidative stress, which can manifest as autoimmune disorders and various cancers.

Trapped Proteins:

- Lymph vessels can become clogged with protein deposits
- Flow can stagnate or even stop for reasons such as fatigue, stress, infection, emotional shock, lack of physical activity, or dehydration
- Results in tissue swelling (edema) accumulated protein in the lymph vessel, along with osmotically held fluids in the interstitial space (lymphedema)
- As toxins accumulate, cells are unable to function properly resulting in various metabolic and infectious problems

Enzyme Therapy:

- **Digestive enzymes** assist proper digestion, thereby impacting the health of the lymphatic system.
- **Lipase** assists in proper fat breakdown and transport to the blood.
- **Digestive enzymes and Probiotics** contribute to the overall health of the gastrointestinal immune system.
- **Proteolytic enzymes** in particular act to restore lymphatic transport capacity.
- **Protease** helps break down the undesired excess proteins that contribute to swelling and inflammation.
- **Proteases** assist in the body's overall circulation and lymphatic flow.
- **Proteolytic enzymes** assist the immune system by toxic removal from organs.

TESTIMONIALS

Re: I'm really happy to have this product on my shelf

"I often use your soothing digestive formula with my clients. I find it to be quite effective especially for people who have a large number of food intolerances, maldigestion or malabsorption. Recently I recommended it for a woman who has fibromyalgia, irritable bowel syndrome, and whose eating options were extremely limited. Along with a probiotic and a few small changes, she is now able to eat a much wider variety of foods without issue. Often I find that the powdered sensitive formula is specifically useful for children and for people who want to begin with just a tiny dose and build up. I'm really happy to have this product on my shelf." - Liz L., PhD, CCN

Re: allow the body to heal itself or optimize well being

"We have used your supplemental digestive enzymes for special needs children evolved over time for the past 15 years... We target patients on the Autistic Spectrum, and any patient who has GI issues. Certainly improving GI flora will help with dysbiosis... Allopathic medicine is not always at the causes and contributing factors of diseases and illness, but tries to fix the symptoms rather than help 'normalize' the terrain/milieu and allow the body to heal itself or to optimize well-being at whatever level of function that may be... As the patient's terrain and gut improve, medication doses might be reduced as absorption is enhanced." - Drs. Pia and Rolf H.

Re: your staph infection protocol did the trick

"The mom of the client that I sent Protease to [4 caps 3xday] just stopped in to say thanks again. It turns out that she had done three rounds of antibiotics and the above protocol did the trick. The infection has completely gone. 'All is well,' she says. 'All healed up and feeling good.'" - Zoe G., BioEnergetics Practitioner

Chapter 10

Cancer: Is It a Deadly Disease?

Cancer persists as a major disease and is afflicting more people today than ever before. Few families remain untouched by this vicious and insidious disease. It is obvious that cancer is a problem, and there are many different theories on it as it continues to grow. It is an accepted belief that cancer cells are formed as a result of physical, infectious, chemical, and genetic mechanisms that interfere with the production of cells. Damaged and abnormal cell production robs the healthy ones of nutrients.

We are told that anyone reading this book could have anywhere from 100 to 300,000 "cancer-like cells" or precancerous cells active in the system right now. Does this mean you have cancer? No, but it does mean you may have unbalanced cells that can behave like cancer. Few people inherit genes that predispose them to cancer (most inherit genes that prevent cancer). Many scientists believe it is genetic, and the answer is in the genes. But if that is the theory, why are there so many suffering from cancer that is not attached to genetics.

I've spent much of my life trying to understand cancer, and I arrived at a conclusion fairly early in the 1960s to 1970s. It is a simplistic view that if the body is undernourished because of poor digestion and absorbing their chemicals inappropriately, a pattern of chronic fatigue and blood-sugar symptoms will manifest. The by-products of improperly digested food in the system block the small and large intestine, causing constipation. This brings on more imposing problems.

Fermentation, putrefaction, and rancidity of partially digested foods take place. Undigested carbohydrates, such as sugars and starch, ferment. Undigested protein putrefies, and undigested fats turn rancid in the intestinal tract. Cancer of any type promotes anaerobic cell activity in putrefied or fermented matter. An anaerobe is a microorganism that can live and grow where there is no free oxygen.

A normal cell multiplies where oxygen is present, but a cancer cell multiplies without oxygen, and this is why they are referred to as acidic cells. These cells are very much at home in an environment of putrefaction and fermentation. Toxins from undigested foods create such an environment. This in turn negatively affects our metabolic balance.

When these conditions prevail, the body sends out signals for help. A group of suitable metabolic enzymes reacts and disintegrates the cancer-like cell. Enzymes carry away toxic debris. New cancer-like cells constantly reproduce, but if we are healthy and balanced, the enzymes can identify and destroy them.

Please understand that if we have a functional immune system coupled with good digestion, our intestines or internal environment should remain disease free. However, if the internal balance is upset by poor eating habits, drugs that weaken the immune system, smoking, stress, premature aging, and living life with fear or anger, we will have an adverse reaction. This happens when the balance between the cancer-like cells and the body's defense systems collapses. Left alone, the cancer-like cells coat themselves with a glue-like protein fiber. This gives them a thickness of 15 times that of normal cells. The cancerous cells hide under the glue in an attempt to remain undetected.

Cancer cells wander through the body, seeking a place where they can anchor themselves. When they do attach to a body part, they rapidly add more of the gluey fiber. This accelerated growth forms a tumor. Cancer cells are both stubborn and clever. They make disguises for themselves called antigens. An antigen is a protein, toxin, or other substance of high molecular weight to which the body reacts by producing antibodies. When the cancer-like cell is destroyed, many times an antigen replaces it. These cells are so persistent that they will even leave a false trail so they can form new antigens elsewhere.

When the antigens become more than our immune system can handle, we are in trouble. When the immune system reaches this depressed state, tissue damage occurs. The cancer cells grow because there is an absence of metabolic enzymes to fight them. In addition, they contain their own enzymatic substance that allows them to multiply at a high rate. Further, they can protect themselves by creating a fibrous coating. The action of protease enzymes strips the fiber coating off the cancer cell. The more of these invaders you have in your body, the more enzymes you need to preserve your health.

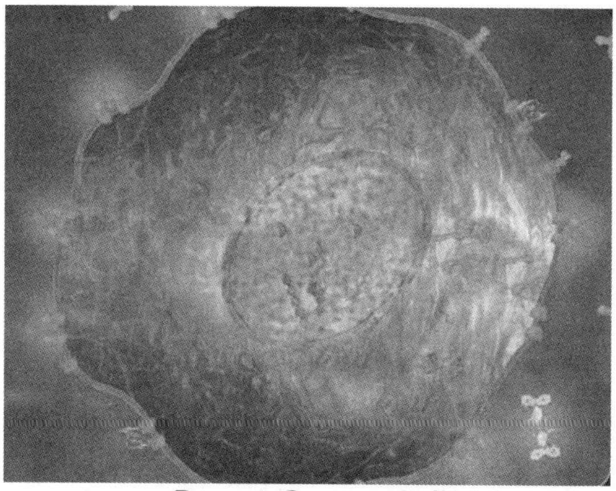

Breast Cancer Cell

I offer you this quotation from Jane Heimlich's book, *What Your Doctor Won't Tell You* (Harper & Row, 1990): "The fiber around the cancer cell is made of protein. Proteolytic enzymes digest this protein coating which allows macrophages (white blood cells) to attack and destroy the cancer cell." In the book *Enzymes: The Fountain of Life,*(written by D.A. Lopez, M.D.; R.M. Williams, M.D.,Ph.D.; and M. Miehlke, M.D.; and published by Neville Press) I quote more doctors' findings: "Cancer cells are able to form imitations of the suckers of certain organs and can therefore adhere to the cells of these organs. The enzymes can apparently differentiate between the true suckers and the imitations by the cancer cells, and can then break away the adhesion molecules, making these proteinaceous counterfeits less of a problem." I grant that even this enzyme book cannot make the final statement on the knowledge of enzymes. Nothing is more stable than change. I conclude by repeating my belief that enzymes represent a highly promising modality of medical treatment. They are the medicines of the future. Their use most surely will increase as we learn more about the immunopathology of diseases through ongoing clinical and scientific studies. I have learned in clinical research that cancer cells are seemingly sensitive to proteolytic enzymes than normal cells.

- Enzymes are known to dissolve the fibrous coating on cancer cells, allowing the immune system to function and to increase better circulation.
- Enzymes play a part in diminishing the ability of cancer cells to attach to healthy tissue.

Your image of cancer will depend on your own perspective. It will depend on if you are the patient, family, friend, or doctor. For me, cancer was an emotional slippery slope. One moment you are encouraged, the next you feel alone, and anger can play a part if you are fearful of the unknown—the "Big C." I personally am not frightened by cancer but why it manifests itself in our bodies.

MY STORY

At the age of 27 I was diagnosed with cancer and set to go into the hospital for a radical hysterectomy. I remember how very anxious, frightened, and victimized when informed of my cancer. Just like everyone, I wanted to know how bad it was, how long I had to live, and what my choices were. I was unprepared for the size of my incision, because of the need to be exploratory; I was cut from hipbone to hipbone. I looked down and the top skin was sewn with wire and baby buttons it looked like all I had to do to see what was inside was to unbutton myself. That really did not concern me as much as some of the follow-up treatments. They left me unable to properly care of my family. We had two children, a daughter and son, who were quite young, and my daughter was continually ill.

I remember finally informing my frustrated oncologist that I simply did not have time for the treatments nor the energy to do so. To me the choices of treatment left me even more worried that I would leave my body before the cancer left it. Instead, I made the choice to treat myself holistically, and this was in the years of Adele Davis (wheat grass and coffee enemas). I tried her theories and was diligent to try most anything that made sense.

One of her quotes: "As I see it, every day you do one of two things: build health or produce disease in yourself." Some things I read just did not make sense to me, but I remained open. Dr. Walker's book about juicing and the toxic colon was an eye opener for me. Juicing for enzymes and nutrients became my mantra, and I juiced everything in sight (a big job) cleaning the vegetables and the juicer. It took dedication, and I stayed away from animal protein. Soon both my daughter and I began losing muscle and became lethargic and weaker. I reintroduced eggs and fish as protein foods, and we began to regain energy.

Receiving the cancer news required a change in my attitude and stress level. I decided my children's lives were more important than my disease. I had to learn how to treat myself with kindness. My intense desire to understand my child's continued poor health was such a driving force to educate myself in all possibilities. After a few years when I was 30 years old and believing all was well in my overall health, I noticed one of my breasts was becoming very itchy deep down inside. In just a few days it was larger than my other breast and kind of red and inflamed looking. I have never feared death, but I had a responsibility to see my children grown.

Rather than have gloom and doom, I worked on mental balance. I am vain, and at 30 years old I was obviously even more so. I did not want anyone cutting my breast off, and I remembered waking up after my first surgery completely unprepared for the size of my incision. So I learned everything I could about this type of cancer. By the way, not much was known about IBC (inflammatory breast cancer) in the 1970s. We know now that Inflammatory Breast Cancer occurs when cancer cells block the lymph vessels in the breast. The blockage causes discoloration or redness, swelling, and warmth. It is a type of cancer, which looks like it grows from the inside of the breast outwards and got pretty ugly and weepy at times.

I personally had witnessed this cancer prior to mine because a dear lady in our church had it, and I watched her struggle with decisions and the ugliness of this type of cancer. She had to pad herself to absorb the matter oozing out of her breast. Treatment today is similar to what was suggested to me back then—chemotherapy, removal of the breast, and radiation. I instead practiced everything I knew from the earlier years, ate the healthiest I knew, and really tried to not dwell on my disappointments in life. My poor oncologist, who was again double frustrated, did recognize that I did have a good response before. However, as he pointed it out to me, it was now back just somewhere else in my body.

In the 1940s there were books written on alkaline versus acid foods, and the idea became popular in the 1970s. The idea is that cancer can only live and grow in an acid cell but cannot survive in an alkaline cell. This confused me after studying food for so many years and earning a degree. However, I tried this for both my child and me. Those foods considered to be alkaline were carbohydrates (vegetables and fruits), and foods considered to be acid were anything from animals (beef, lamb, pig, fowl, and fish). I was always interested in blood rheology so I studied with the Darkfield microscope and felt that I would see the difference if this was indeed possible. In the labs I had already used a bright-field lens and different microscopes, but they required stained, dead, or smeared blood samples but never living blood samples. With this new tool, I would suggest clients to eat these alkaline foods and see if it affected their blood by taking a small sample of blood and observing it. Then by making further changes in their diet, I would look to see if there was a change in the blood and questionnaire—doing the same with nutrients to invoke change and looking to see if there was a change in the plasma. All this only led me to question the acid/alkaline diet and have even more questions about digestion. I simply was not seeing what I should, if what they surmised was true.

Once again I began to go back into the extreme fatigue we suffered during our juicing period. I bought different types of medical mushrooms, let them sit to give off enzyme-healing properties, and I would drink the fluid it brewed. Listen when you are facing leaving your children, you will do most anything no matter how bad it tastes! But try we did until my cancer spread to another organ. I finally recognized that it was up to me to make our decisions that made sense and to fight back. No one else could do it for me. I just needed to know how to do it. We did not have computers or the Internet, so it was books, classes, and trial and error. Actually I'm happy there wasn't the Internet, or I would have become even more confused.

This time I made it to my 35th birthday when bloody stools appeared with some lower abdominal pain; much like when I was a child. The "Big C" had moved into my large intestine (colon). I kept to my regimen or should say, went back to it. Like so many, when I thought I was healthy, I started back to old habits. But when finding out I was not healthy, I jumped back to what I needed to do. I added another validation testing since I was still confused about how different foods, whether acid or alkaline, influenced a cell change.

I learned the Dr. Carey Reams Testing. Others have taken it up and given it different names, but it is the same theory and basically the same testing using his mathematical numbers. This was interesting to me because I could take our urine and saliva, and by adding different reagents or checking pH papers, it gave me various results marking our biochemical health. He had mathematical results that were to indicate the proper balance for the environment of a human. If I had an opinion, it was the use of random urine rather that a 24-hour catch, but I still found it useful. Dr. Reams tested our fluids as he would the soil. He was an agriculturist and a practitioner that understood the link of health. A friend of mine that has passed by the name of Dean Stonier was the first person to introduce me to him. There were diets and nutrients you ingested according to the results of your urine and saliva. Dr. M.T. Morter expanded on this work and is still teaching it today.

Nevertheless, during my seven years of dealing with cancer, I knew without a doubt we are much more than just our bodies or our minds, but we are also our spirits. They make up who we are, and to focus on just one does not allow for balance. I looked at every part of my life because I know many diseases are a wake-up call and an opportunity to look deeper into our beliefs and negative emotions. I've learned that this is a time to focus inside us and not outside ourselves. I loved studying this and concentrating on how the body works and what we do to sabotage ourselves whether it is in our health or our emotions. It was during my third bout of cancer I discovered supplemental digestive enzymes for my daughter's illness. We both got on them, and I focused on the proteases between meals since it just made sense to me. This is back at the beginning when protease enzymes formulated by Dr. Howell were only just above 16,000 units of protease activity in a capsule, and I had to take from 50 to 75 capsules a day. We did not have anything to go by back then, but I used tests to see how many I seemed to require. Obviously, I got to know his company and eventually taught for them because I was free of cancer and knew the value of enzymes. It has been 35 years, and I am still free of cancer.

Do I believe in bringing balance to the body so it can heal itself? Absolutely. Do I feel that supplemental digestive enzymes helped me save my life? Yes, without a doubt. Do I suggest that others take enzymes to bring life to the body? Yes. However, I never pressure anyone to do or take something they do not believe in themselves. If they feel comfortable with the guidance of their doctors, I will honor that. It is not my place to try to force anyone to follow my program.

All individuals have the right to make their own decisions about how they wish to handle their own health. No one else has that right and cannot do it for them. It is up to all of us to educate ourselves and make our choices based on knowledge and belief, rather than fear and coercion. I am the first to say that enzymes are not the only answer to good health. Nevertheless, the one thing we all must do to rebuild and heal is feed and fortify through efficient digestion. Every food we consume has to be digested, assimilated, and utilized as fuel if we want to continually make new, vital cells.

Good news! I've formulated a blend of systemic proteolytic enzymes and the capsule contains over 400,000 HUT of Proteases. Someone like myself would take only 12 capsules a day to arrive at the amount I tried for back in the days of my cancer when I took 50 to 75 capsules a day.

I mentioned cleaning up our beliefs, practice forgiveness, and treat yourself with love or kindness. I wrote about what I know about supplemental plant-based enzymes to meet insufficient enzyme needs for health. Now it is time to speak of nutrition. I refer you to the Renewal Program chapter and its information on how to renew your health.

Back in the 1960s onward I started a program for different biochemical individuals to know what foods give them energy and which ones cause an imbalance. I knew that sugar was not good for anyone and since I have an added problem breaking down carbohydrates, it was very real to me. I recognized that I personally did very well on diets similar to Dr. Adkins', and when I tried to consume the foods I craved, I felt unwell. Those carbohydrate foods were all high in sugar.

During the same time I was looking for answers, several physicians and scientists began to come up with a theory about cancer. The road to the cancer front has been littered with major breakthroughs that never materialized into breakthrough solutions. Through these many years the struggle goes on. However, there has been enough work in nutrition regulating glucose. Glucose feeds cancer cells. It became clear how tumors escape many so-called cancer therapies. Cancer cells will escape as long as they can maintain their ability to ferment. If cancer cells cannot ferment, they will die. Uncontrolled cell growth is driven by insufficient respiration (lack of oxygen) with compensatory fermentation. Fermentation is a metabolic process converting sugars to acids. Hence the saying, sugar feeds cancer or the acidic cancer cell.

They suggest keeping your glucose range down so that the fat cells can be burned for energy.

If you want more detailed cancer information I refer you to *Cancer as a Metabolic Disease* by Dr. Thomas N. Seyfried. The book is on the origin, management, and prevention of cancer. It can be found on Amazon and is offered in the Kindle edition. It contains pictures of different types of cancers, but it is a detailed scientific book.

I started this chapter with the title: CANCER: IS IT A DEADLY DISEASE?

Here are a few facts from just one year (latest information from the year 2010):

- Breast Cancer killed around 40,170 women in 2010
- Lung and Bronchus Cancer killed around 159,390 persons in 2010
- Colon and Rectum Cancer killed around 49,920 persons in 2010
- Skin Cancer killed around 11,590 persons in 2010
- Brain and Nervous System Cancer killed around 12,920 persons 2010
- Liver and Bile Duct Cancer killed around 18,910 people
- Compare the above numbers to 32,885 car crash fatalities in 2010

These are just a few of the more than 150 different types of cancer.

See "The Seven Stages of Disease" chapter on how we create our own conditions.

CANCER MYTHS

This topic has been a real concern to me as I have seen and read an increasing amount of misinformation on cancer in magazine articles, books, and the media. Now that we are in an age of instant information located on the Internet, there is often confusion between what is correct and incorrect. Do I believe I have all the answers? I will be very honest and say no. However, I am a cancer survivor for over 30 years and have spent many years studying the complexity of the human system to better understand how a human being physically operates.

That's why my heart goes out to so many who are desperate for good information. Many think because if it's in a book, it has to be true; or if written by a health practitioner, it has to be accurate. When in truth, much is uneducated thoughts or theories. I use the word "theory" because it means it is an idea, but not scientifically proven or possible. As a believer in education, I am hoping to bring these myths to the forefront and through education help you learn to identify truth for the human's system.

MYTH—CANCER CELLS THRIVE IN AN ACID ENVIRONMENT BUT CANNOT THRIVE IN AN ALKALINE ENVIRONMENT

Should someone with cancer avoid eating animal products? Some experts endorse a diet made of 80 percent fresh vegetables, juice, whole grains, seeds, nuts, and a little fruit to help put the body into an alkaline environment. About 20 percent can be from cooked food, including beans. However, all meat, fowl, or fish are considered acidic, and it is claimed they will result in causing our cells to become acid if consumed.

Let's start with the digestive system to best understand how this theory can simply not be true. Since this is about acid versus alkaline foods, you will need to know what acid or alkaline pH means. Put simply, anything with a pH of 6.9 or below is considered acidic; 7.0 is neutral; and alkaline means anything 7.1 or above. This will become clearer as you consider each of the major digestive organs.

STOMACH

- All food that has been chewed and/or swallowed goes into the stomach. An empty stomach remains slightly acidic (5.0 pH) when empty.
- As food enters the stomach (no matter if it is vegetables, fruits, fats, or meats) it begins to send out signals for more acids in order to break down the proteins in all food.
- These stomach acids create a very acidic environment down to (1.5 pH).
- If we have a healthy stomach, the mucosal lining of the stomach protects it from the extreme acids being produced.
- This is where all protein is broken down for proper digestion by protease enzymes.

- Because Vitamin B12 and some minerals require protein breakdown to liberate them from the food, this is where those nutrients are acquired.
- Food remains in the stomach anywhere from three to five hours while being properly broken down. (When people mention they feel like food is still in their stomach after they've eaten – they may be correct!)
- The time spent in the stomach will depend on the contents of the foods eaten.
- The end result is called bolus and consists of partially digested food, water, acid, and digestive enzymes.

SMALL INTESTINE

- This food-acid-enzyme mixture then squirts into the duodenum (first part of small intestine) and mixes with bicarbonate from the pancreas and the alkaline bile from the gallbladder, which is necessary for breakdown of fats.
- Bile raises the acid bolus (now referred to as chyme) out of the extreme acid into a neutral pH of 7.0.
- At a pH of 7, the acid-based enzymes that were present from the stomach are no longer active. This then leads into the further breakdown of the nutrients still present by anaerobic bacteria, which at the same time help synthesize vitamin B and vitamin K.
- This neutral or slightly alkaline small intestine environment calls on the pancreas for carbohydrate-splitting digestive enzymes to finalize the digestion of carbohydrates (vegetables, grains, starch, and fruits).
- The lymphatic system residing inside the small intestine takes the emulsified fats (broken down by lipase enzymes) and transfers them into the blood where they are taken to the liver to be broken down into cholesterol or stored.
- The rest of the chyme (semifluid mass of partially-digested food without fats) are moved through the small intestine which contains muscle moving the chyme along, and its villi (hair-like projections) absorbs water-soluble vitamins and amino acids from the broken down proteins.

Please understand that this process, just as the one through the stomach, takes another four to five hours before it moves into the large intestine.

LARGE INTESTINE / COLON

- Final stage of digestion where the useless waste ends up.
- The colon is slightly shorter than the small intestine at 4.9 feet long but wider and in an acidic range.
- The large intestine houses over 700 species of bacteria that perform several important functions. One important function is to produce a large amount of vitamins such as Vitamin K, Vitamin B3, and other important B vitamins.
- Food is no longer broken down at this stage, however the absorption of vitamins created by the colon bacteria is necessary for our health.
- The healthy bacteria also produce antibodies (immune fighters) for the foods that are causing problems during digestion.
- Bacteria can also produce gas from the improperly broken down carbohydrates and fiber.
- The large intestine takes about at least 16 hours or more to finish the process of the digestive system.

In a healthy adult, the process of digestion from one meal alone can take anywhere from 24 to 72 hours. This will vary between individuals and as a result of the size of the meal. Other factors that CAN hinder digestion include medication, constipation, and use of antibiotics, because all of these cause problems with the bacteria strains.

Digestion is a complex process, and pH certainly plays a very crucial role in a normal functioning digestive tract. However, the pH of the individual foods does NOT significantly sway the digestive environment as a whole. Therefore, it cannot affect the acidity of the cells either.

Acid pH is any number that is below 7.0 pH and alkaline is any number above 7.0 pH. If foods themselves were able to influence the cells with acid or alkaline, more than likely, you would not be around to read this book. What I mean by this statement is that to be alive and healthy our blood must remain slightly alkaline at all times. Our blood cells needs to stay within a narrow range of 7.34 to 7.45 pH, or our heart will stop beating. Your digestive system remains more acid to neutral pH, or you would become very ill. Every organ has its own specific healthy pH.

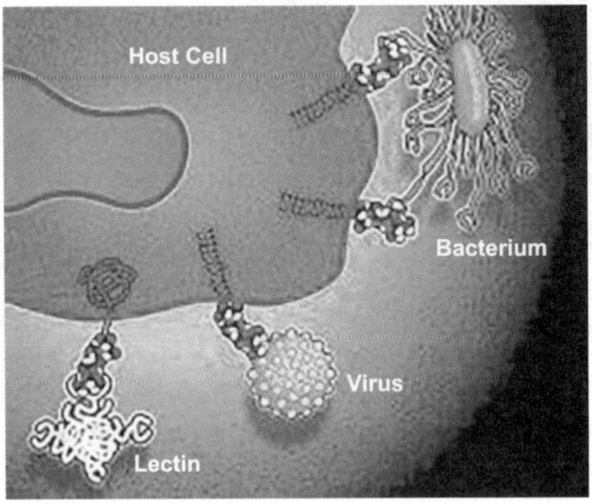

ACID OR ALKALINE ASH DIET

To be very honest with you, I need to disclose that the reason I spent years at the Universities, and ended up with the education I now have, was truly driven by these impossible theories. I literally had to go to school to determine what was possible or detrimental. I had cancer and a sick child, and it was if it were life and death. Like Susan Powter I wanted to scream, "Stop the Insanity!" I tried so many things because when you are desperate, you will do almost anything.

Please, do not let terminology (technical applications) confuse you. The nutrition world tends to misinterpret information and then use ambiguous (double meaning or unclear) statements, creating confusion especially when they are not scientifically grounded.

SEPARATING THE FACTS FROM THE FADS

The Internet can be very misleading. I saw one site that read, "Acid blood kills and alkaline blood lives." Actually when out of homeostasis, they both can kill. The body is very sensitive to its pH level, so strong mechanisms exist to maintain it. Outside the acceptable pH range, proteins are denatured and enzymes lose their ability to function and death occurs. Your stomach is so acidic that no food can change its acidity. Citrus fruits, vinegar, and vitamins such as ascorbic acid (vitamin C) or folic acid do not change the acidity of your stomach or your bloodstream. No "foods" change the acidity or alkalinity of anything in your body. Foods, however, may affect the urine with color or smell such as asparagus.

There are four medical terms for this acid versus alkaline process. They are metabolic acidosis, respiratory acidosis, metabolic alkalosis, and respiratory alkalosis. One or a combination may occur at any given time. Respiratory or kidney failure is the end result. For example, when you hold your breath, carbon dioxide accumulates in your bloodstream very rapidly and your blood turns acidic, and you will become uncomfortable or even pass out. This forces you to start breathing again immediately, and the pH returns to normal. If your kidneys are damaged and cannot regulate the acidity of your bloodstream, chemical reactions stop, poisons accumulate in your bloodstream, and you can die. Alkalosis can be caused from severe vomiting, diarrhea, and the loss of potassium and water. Some medical drugs, pneumonia, or any oxygenation problem can negatively influence our respiratory system. These are the things that influence the blood, not foods.

One of my PhDs that I earned was in dietetics and in the process we learned about food ash. This was the study analysis of food ash and mineral content. Foods burn to ash in a specialized oven (muffle oven), which maintains high temperatures over 600 degrees. This is done to measure the foods nutrient (mineral) content and started years ago, but it still goes on today for some food labeling and quality assurance. Obviously, we humans do not have an internal oven which burns the foods we eat into ash, nor do our enzymes cause a combustible heat that turns the food you eat into ash. Yet, some people believe when we eat we can metabolize our food into ash and by some magical unknown it goes on to influence our blood. It is just not humanly possible.

Am I against eating foods that are considered alkaline? Absolutely not! They are plant foods, and we need them just as much as we need good fats and healthy proteins. I spent years studying food nutrition and Health Science and personally believe organic fresh vegetables and fruits (foods free of GMOs) along with grass-fed beef, wild fish, and fowl (free from injected hormones) is necessary for life. Foods heal, not because they are alkaline or acid, but because they provide nourishment for growth and the maintenance of life.

DOES SUGAR REALLY CAUSE CANCER?

One of the biggest driving forces in disease is sugar. We should not consume sugar and yet most crave it. Sugar is actually the demon that changes or prepares a cell for cancer. Is it a food? They call it a carbohydrate and a food. But is it? Sugar is chemically extracted from sugar beets or sugar cane and refined into simple sugar.

Sugar MIXED IN FOOD does not have the ability nor magically goes directly into a cell.

The overconsumption of carbohydrates along with simple sugars compromises the liver and pancreas. It is actually the glucose these foods breakdown into. It then is used for metabolism.

Metabolism is the process your body uses to get or make energy from the food you eat. Food is made up of proteins, carbohydrates, and fats. Chemicals in your digestive system break the food parts down into glucose, fatty acids and amino acids, your body's fuel. Your body can use this fuel right away, or it can store the glucose in your body tissues, such as your liver, muscles, and body fat. Amino acids cannot be stored.

A metabolic disorder occurs when abnormal chemical reactions in your body disrupt this process. When this happens, you might have too much of some substances or too little of other ones that you need to stay healthy. You can develop a metabolic disorder when some organs, such as your liver or pancreas, become diseased or do not function normally. Diabetes is an example. There is a large body of science that proves Cancer is a Metabolic Disease, and the large amount of glucose causes cancer and allows it to multiply.

Here lies the oxymoron or contradiction of alkaline food theory—all fruit and vegetables, which are called "alkaline," are broken down to glucose and dependent on your own personal metabolic condition. This can be good or bad.

SUGAR IN BEVERAGES MAY HAVE THE ABILITY TO GO DIRECTLY TO THE CELL.

A study has gone on since 1986 involving 23,039 postmenopausal women. Maki Inoue-Choi, Ph.D., M.S., R.D., led this study as a research associate in the Division of Epidemiology and Community Health of the University of Minnesota School of Public Health in Minneapolis.

Men, please do not mistakenly assume that only postmenopausal women can have this sugar-driven cancer problem. They just happen to be the group studied since there has been an alarming rise in endometrial cancers amongst postmenopausal women. To be honest, there has been a marked rise in testicular and prostate cancer in men as well.

Choi and colleagues used dietary intake from postmenopausal women's demographic information and medical history, prior to the cancer diagnosis, as part of the Iowa Women's Health Study.

Postmenopausal women who consume sugar-sweetened beverages are more likely to develop the most common type of endometrial cancer compared with women who do not drink sugar-sweetened beverages, according to a study published in *Cancer Epidemiology, Biomarkers & Prevention*, a journal of the American Association for Cancer Research.

Postmenopausal women who reported the highest intake of sugar-sweetened beverages had a 78 percent increased risk for estrogen-dependent type I endometrial cancer (the most common type of this disease). The more sugar-sweetened beverages a woman drank, the higher her risk.

As reported in the study, a questionnaire from Harvard included questions asking usual intake frequency of sugar-sweetened beverages:

(1) Coke®, Pepsi®, or other colas with sugar

(2) Caffeine-free Coke®, Pepsi®, or other colas with sugar

(3) Other carbonated beverages with sugar (e.g., 7-Up®)

(4) Hawaiian Punch®, lemonade, or other non-carbonated fruit drinks

(5) Sugar-free soft drinks, including low-calorie caffeinated and caffeine-free Cola (e.g., Diet-Coke®, Pepsi-Free®), and other low-calorie carbonated beverages (e.g., Fresca®, Diet 7-Up®, and Diet Ginger Ale®)

The questionnaire included baked goods and other forms of sugary foods but the beverage turned out to be the concern. *"One theory is that sugar from whole foods come with other nutrients, fat (and) fiber, so they may slow sugar absorption," Choi said.*

Please see the chapter on "The Seven Stages of Disease." Hopefully, I will be able to make it clear once and for all time that we are responsible for our own health.

Chapter 11

The Seven Stages of Disease

It has been my experience to witness fear, surprise, and utter confusion by a person receiving a negative diagnosis. Disease is never supposed to happen to us. We believe that this condition happened to us overnight, and there was absolutely nothing that could have been done to spare us. Many of us feel like victims and completely without choice in this matter. I have been in this position more than once in my lifetime and understand the fear and feeling of helplessness. However, what I have since learned is there are choices, and most conditions do not happen overnight. The choices a person makes not to ever exercise, or to stop for lunch every day and eat fast foods, or lead a stressful, negative lifestyle that can lead to the depletion and an imbalance of enzymes. Every one of us is born with an inherited ability to make metabolic enzymes. However, enzymes can either be repressed or destroyed when the body's condition or environment is not in balance.

It is these poor choices that we make. In fact, they result in the imbalances to the whole body, which allows disease to manifest. No, disease does not happen overnight. It takes years of this constant neglect and over-indulgence to alter our metabolic enzyme balance and create a disease condition. I wrote this many years ago for my thesis when I decided to quit studying disease and switched my degree from an M.D. to a Ph.D. in Health Sciences. My focus was on how a body works when in balance. By that I could then track ahead to the nature of a disease process. There are many cancer survivors like myself and there are things we have in common. One is education about our disease in order to stop our movement down that cancer slippery slope we were riding on. We did not want it to ride right into another organ and set up residence there. I hope you will recognize yourself in one of the stages and plan a way back to a healthier stage and into quality of life.

STAGE ONE

This stage is characterized by approximately 95 percent lifestyle and/or environmental factors.

The first phase of imbalance can be caused by overeating, drinking, overwork, worry and over-indulgence in processed food. Foods that are processed lack the nutrients to assist in your cell health. Our metabolic enzymes that are produced by our organs on demand are limited. Stress and alcohol deplete valuable enzymes. Sugar, salt, caffeine, soft drinks, tobacco, drugs, serum injections, impure water, polluted air, tension, depression, and lack of rest only add to the extra burden for the body to produce the necessary enzymes required for good health. The result is a weakened immune system and reduced vital energy or strength. How many of us choose to do this on a regular basis and never stop to think about the outcome?

In this stage our metabolic enzymes (biochemically produced in the body) have now become compromised. Even the simplest efforts of the body like mastication (chewing to begin the first step of digestion and increasing the surface area of foods to allow more efficient breakdown by enzymes). Receiving the proper enzyme support is now limited. If we could aid the body by adding supplemental plant-based digestive enzyme supplements such as proteases to help break down the proteins; carbohydrate-splitting enzymes to break down the carbohydrates and starch; and lipase to break down the fats; we have at least begun to help the body regain its balance.

Etiology:

Beginning of malnutrition is overwhelmingly the result of poor lifestyle choices and environmental factors. Weakened immune response reduced vital energy, metabolic digestive enzymes compromised, and the impairment of the digestive system.

Recommendations:

- Improve food choices according to your Biochemical Type
- Drink at least six 10-ounce glasses of pure water each day
- Start a regular exercise program in order to alleviate stress
- Mentally appreciate what you have while looking for joy in your life
- Possible three to six week program dependent on compliance to diet change and ingesting the digestive enzymes at meals

Supplement Recommendations:

- Supplemental plant-based digestive enzymes; 1-2 caps with each meal and snack

Protocol if starting a new exercise program:

- Supplemental plant-based systemic protease; 2-3 caps following exercise for inflammation

STAGE TWO

The choices above when not corrected will progressively overwhelm the system and create this next stage:

The second phase is created when the body's ability has become so compromised it cannot even properly digest food. Result—there is an increase in food toxins. The initial lack of enzymes, created by the first stage, has slowed down the elimination of toxins by the liver and kidneys and has placed a burden on the body's defense system.

Poor nutrition from Phase One did not provide the necessary elements to supply the body's building blocks for metabolic enzymes, antibodies, and even hormones, and free radicals have taken their toll. These factors can be accentuated with age as the body accumulates various toxins, which provides a continuous weakening.

During digestion, a lot of blood must flow to the digestive organs. Energies of the system are always divided between assimilation and elimination. An unequal use of those energies is again created by the practice of overeating, and the other abusive choices mentioned in stage one. Science tells us that we use 80 to 90 percent of the body's energies just digesting food alone. Other stimulating choices also divert energy. The stimulating foods as an example are caffeine, sodas, sugars, and alcohol. When non-usable substances and their toxins are not or cannot be eliminated, they are stored in the tissues, joints, and organs. This leaves the body intoxicated, sluggish, and weakened. One of the recognizable signs may be constipation, but there are other signs of toxicity that begin here.

Now the body is not only overburdened with toxins, but the struggle of the body's enzymatic potential to keep up the proper digestive enzymes, hormones, rebuild muscle, tissue, bone, etc. is now impaired. A sluggish, continually tired body is susceptible to crises. Simple over-the-counter digestive aids do not work here. It takes supplemental plant-based digestive enzymes to replenish proper digestion to the body. Other chemically based substances will only add toxicity to the body.

Obviously, the supplemental digestive enzymes mentioned in stage one need to be increased with meals.

Etiology:

The natural progression of toxic removal by the body is now hindered.

Continued poor choices progressively overwhelm the system. Metabolic digestive enzymes continue to decrease; digestive system becomes sluggish, slowing elimination of toxins.

Recommendations:

- Address food choices according to your Biochemical Type
- Monitor exercise program
- Increasing digestive enzymes is a necessity
- Simple over-the-counter digestive aids are just a bandage, plus chemically-based substances will add toxicity to the already burdened system
- Cut back on the amount of sugar eaten
- Avoid sugar substitutes
- Avoid improper fat consumption or trans-fatty acids (hidden fats)
- Drink enough water for a healthy cell
- Control stress with simple deep breathing techniques
- Possible 9 to 12 week program to create balance

Supplement recommendations:

- Supplemental plant-based digestive enzymes; 2-3 with meals
- Systemic protease first thing in AM and before bed
- Probiotic before bed

Constipation and/or Leaky Gut are in this stage. Adjust probiotics to assist in elimination.

STAGE THREE

Progression to stage three involves the pH imbalances and a definite deterioration to the biological chemistry. Cellular energy is compromised.

To best explain Biological Chemistry is to think of the correlation between our environment (both outside the body and inside the body) and disease. Biological chemistry inside the body refers to the environment that surrounds the cells of our bodies. It contains the fluids, the nutrients, the minerals and trace elements, adjoining cells of all our systems, plus a host of both good and bad microorganisms. If that seems a bit overwhelming, try and picture our red blood cells suspended by our plasma (a clear fluid), which is full of nutrients but can also include bacteria, parasites, yeasts, and fat globules. Our white blood cells or Immune cells are referred to as plasma cells. When I look at live blood in my microscope I am observing these very things.

The third stage represents an increased acidity in the plasma. Energy at the cell is now being hindered. When continual poor eating and drinking habits are repeated, it leads to over-acid plasma. Once this plasma saturates our cells, we will experience a loss of electrons (energy) from the cell itself. Potassium, chlorides, magnesium and other minerals, along with our life's energy, will then be carried out of the body via the kidneys.

This biochemical imbalance further impairs our metabolic system, our lungs' respiration rate, and digestive ability. This is because the digestive system cannot produce the signal for hydrochloric acid in the stomach for digestion. The absence of free hydrochloric acid in the stomach leads to chronic gastritis. The burping, belching, and gas that can result from these chronic problems can again be alleviated by the use of supplemental digestive enzymes. Over-the-counter antacids only increase this problem, because remember, the body's number one priority is to keep the system in balance. If we add alkaline substances, the body will create acid to sustain its balance, and the cycle becomes repeated over and over. This stage calls for enough supplemental digestive enzymes with meals and between meals to meet these stage requirements. Probiotics in this stage are as necessary as are proteases.

Etiology:

A ratio of ions and electrical charges in the cell become imbalanced.

You now are experiencing deterioration of the body's internal environment and imbalances caused by increased toxicity in the body. These results make up the third stage.

Recommendations:

- Diet and lifestyle improvements according to Biochemical Type
- Eliminate all soft drinks and regulate coffee consumption

- Eliminate all synthetic sugars
- Drink adequate pure water (six to eight 10-ounce glasses) for kidney balance
- Walking exercise to improve breathing
- Replace good bacteria with probiotics
- Make sure there is adequate rest for healing
- Possible three to four month program dependent on consistency

Supplement recommendations:

- Increase digestive enzymes with meals
- Increase probiotics before bed and possibly first thing in AM
- Increase systemic protease; 2 capsules, 3 times a day (one cap = 400,000 HUT)

Or choose symptoms below for protocols:

- Fatigue
- Mineral Imbalances – Potassium and Magnesium
- Organ assistance – Kidney Drainage or Lymphatic Drainage
- Panic attacks – Soothing remedy to calm
- Heavy Metal Detox Protocol
- Hyperlipidemia Protocol
- Constipation Protocol
- Allergy Protocol
- Asthma Protocol

STAGE FOUR

The continuances of constant toxicity have created a depressed environment and symptoms increase. Inflammation, which is normal to the body, is now becoming more chronic and is a constant recurring problem that is becoming difficult to eradicate.

This stage coincides with further deterioration of the metabolic environment (presence of high levels of toxins). Various parasitic and pathogenic growth factors continue invading the body:

- There is an accumulation of metabolic wastes, which includes dead cells
- The inability of the waste removal system to adjust to the load now being imposed on it
- Increased growth of bad bacteria over beneficial bacteria
- Accumulation of toxic materials within the organs, joints, and other vital parts of the body become apparent
- Death of our 25 trillion red blood cells alone, seven million die per second and their by-products contain toxins such as carbon dioxide
- Anabolism (healthy growth) is greatly affected and emphasis of the body's cellular activity is directed to defense
- Additionally, the buffering capacity of the body fluids is impaired
- Series of symptoms manifested by stone-like formations in the joints, kidneys, and gall bladder, which consist of trapped inorganic substances from poorly digested food, drink, and/or drugs may be noted

These toxic substances are indigestible, but at the same time, cannot be expelled by the weakened body system. For example, so-called "allergies" may be nothing more than the irritation of already chronically inflamed nasal passages from a pronounced toxemic condition. Toxemia is the basic cause of inflammation, including the lining of the membranes of the hollow organs of the body. Heat, redness, swelling, and pain are characterized in this stage.

Science has now proven that all allergies, whether airborne or food, begins in the gut. 80 percent of our immune system resides inside the digestive tract. With the body's immune state being compromised, additional supplemental protease now becomes a vital supplement for the body to survive these attacks. Protease not only becomes critical to the digestion of important proteins in the digestive tract, but will also bind to alpha 2-macroglobulin and delivered to the sites of immune function. Years of clinical experience have shown that toxins are also removed from the blood, perhaps from an overall improvement in blood flow. The circulation and improved blood flow begins with additional supplemental protease taken between meals. In addition, protease supplemental digestive enzymes taken with meals provides for a very high level of antioxidants between meals along with probiotics taken at bedtime.

Etiology:

Chronic Inflammation: These continued high levels of body toxicity create a contaminated physical environment, and inflammation throughout the body becomes very chronic. Digestion abilities have a slower transit time.

Recommendations:

- Balanced diet with several small meals—more like grazing during the day
- Walk twice a day for 20 minutes on a daily basis
- Adequate fluids and rest
- Possible 6-month program dependent on compliance

Supplement recommendations:

- Supplemental plant-based digestive enzymes with each meal and snack
- Supplemental Protease with the meal
- At least 6 caps or more systemic (2 capsules, 3 times a day) is needed.
- Probiotic 2 times a day

Or choose symptoms below for correct supplementation:

- Anemia Protocol
- Allergy Protocol
- Candida Protocol
- Fibromyalgia / CFS Protocol
- Arthritis Protocol
- Inflammation Protocol
- Eczema Protocol
- Psoriasis Protocol
- Rosacea Protocol
- Gastroesophageal Reflux Protocol
- Headache-Cluster Protocol
- Headaches-Tension Protocol
- Headaches-Migraine Protocol
- IBS Protocol
- Gallbladder Stress Protocol
- Toxicity Protocol
- Anxiety Protocol
- Asthma Protocol
- Hypoglycemia Protocol

- Adrenal and/or thyroid conditions

STAGE FIVE

This stage constitutes the onset of the actual disease due to organ deterioration and functional impairment. Chronic inflammation is characterized by the beginning of tissue destruction.

The fifth phase of degeneration is characterized by further weakening of the body, frequent recurrence of ailments, and "disease" onset. This is when a gradual thickening (hardening) of the mucous and sub-mucous tissue takes place. This is due to the causes of chronic inflammation, which remain unchanged from the last stage. This increased level of hardening chokes arterial circulation (hardening of the arteries), cutting off oxygen and the food supply. The tissues clump and break down, giving rise to skin disorders. These skin problems can be skin eruptions such as moles, liver spots, callused feet, and other dead cell accumulations. The lymphatic system becomes stagnate, is unable to utilize antioxidants, and puts the body in oxidative stress and premature tissue aging. At this point, any metabolic digestive enzymes the body has to supply for digestion is completely limited by the condition of the body. Many suffer from indigestion, bloating, gas, and burning sensations in the gastrointestinal area.

Definition:

Pathological process having characteristic set of signs and symptoms. It may affect the whole body or any of its parts, and its ideology, pathology, and prognosis may be known or unknown.

Etiology:

The possibility of an actual disease may take place in this phase. Basis of internal inflammation has not been changed; outwardly obvious signs and symptoms of health problems are now evident. Women become aware of their hormonal imbalances. This is the stage many will "finally" seek care.

Recommendations:

- Lymphatic Massage
- Nutritional consultation for lifestyle change is necessary to rebuild cells and adequate protein for rebuilding
- Walk 2-3 times a day to get oxygen to the cell
- Adequate water and rest for stress control

- Hormonal screening
- Consider "The Renewal Diet"
- Possible 6 to 9 month program dependent on compliance

Supplemental recommendations:

- Supplemental plant-based digestive enzymes with all food
- Additional protease with the foods
- Probiotics possibly with each meal or three times per day
- Chronic Inflammation—Systemic protease several times a day
- Hormonal Imbalances—Feed and Fortify Adrenal and Thyroid

Or choose symptoms below for correct supplementation:

- Diabetes Protocol
- Skin Rejuvenation Protocol
- GERD Protocol
- Peptic Ulcers Protocol
- Gout Protocol
- Adrenal Protocol
- Menopause Protocol
- Osteopenia Protocol
- Celiac Disease Protocol
- Hypertension Protocol
- Periodontal Protocol
- Lupus Protocol
- Lymphedema Protocol
- Menière's Disease Protocol
- Hemorrhoid Protocol
- Precancerous conditions
- Shingles
- Hypoglycemia

STAGE SIX

The ability of the body has now given way to degenerative diseases and major system dysfunction occurs. For instance, instead of normal toxin elimination, excretion of toxic-laden mucus erupts from open wounds, boils, fistulas, internal ulcers, chancre (as in AIDS), and herpes simplex. These excretions can occur from the eyes, ears, nose, vagina, or other body cavities. Other symptoms in this stage could be high or low blood sugar and/or anorexia, which are nothing more than SHS (sugar handling stress) due to adrenal exhaustion from a highly toxic condition. Irritable bowel syndrome and ulcerated states are now seen in this stage. The good and bad bacteria in the colon are now out of balance, and the bad bacteria are striving to take over the enzyme sights of the villi in our intestines. The overgrowth of the bad bacteria fight for control of the same sights so they can eat off of the poorly-digested food sources. The ability of the body to breakdown wheat or other grains at this stage is further handicapped by the overgrowth of bad bacteria.

Conditions at this stage will worsen. Indigestion/malabsorption will favor the overgrowth of undesirable and opportunistic micro-flora in the GI tract, which will convert the poorly digested foods into toxic compounds, many of them shown to induce cancer. For instance, studies have shown that excess cholesterol may be converted by some undesirable bacteria of the GI micro-flora into estrogen-like compounds that are cancer promoting: thus in addition to any normal estrogen produced by the body as normal physiological process, more estrogen may be produced by poor digestion creating an excess imbalance in the body.

Microorganisms (good and bad bacteria) are out of balance, and the undesirable bacteria of the micro-flora begin promoting cancer like cells and undesirable cancer causing hormones.

Probiotic supplementation ("friendly" bacteria) now has become not just preventative, but a necessity for the health of the whole. A preferred probiotic that should be part of your probiotic formula is Lactobacillus plantarum (l. plantarum) with the ability to eliminate or reduce most other bad bacteria and fungi as it is the dominating habitat of all sorts of naturally-fermented foods. L. plantarum has an up-regulatory effect on the immune system, changes the immune cells, and influences production of cytokines. One consequence of this is the normalization of the colon pH.

Etiology:

Cellular starvation and disease progressive state: Degenerative diseases and major system dysfunction have reached critical levels. Instead of normal toxin elimination you now have eruptions or excretions of toxic laden mucous such as open wounds, boils, fistulas, internal ulcers and herpes simplex. Other symptoms in this stage are hormonal involvements such as imbalance of insulin.

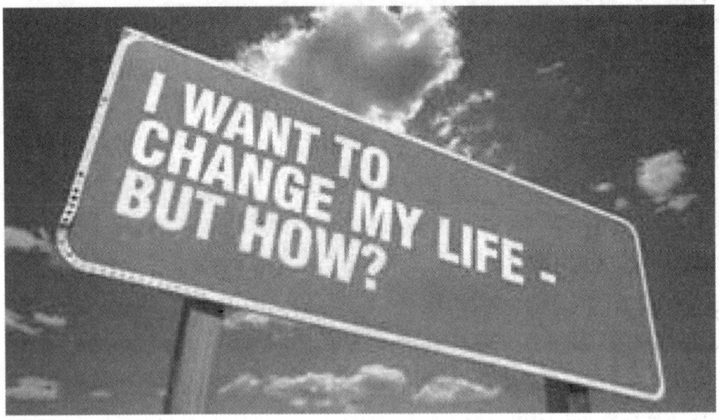

Recommendations:

- Besides the lifestyle changes a psychological workup is necessary
- Renewal Program defines exercise (only walking) on a daily basis
- Eat 3-4 ounces of protein with vegetables every 3.5 to 4 hours, up to 6 times a day
- Adequate fluid intake (6-8 glasses pure water), sleep, and stress control
- Quiet time in a healthy environment
- If menopausal, test hormones and assess their Menopausal Type or Andropause
- Possible nine to 12-month program dependent on compliance and condition

Supplemental recommendations:

- Supplemental plant-based digestive enzymes (it now depends on kind and strength)
- Supplemental protease in addition at meals
- Systemic protease needs to be increased to at least 8 capsules daily (2 caps, 4 times a day)
- Probiotics must be increased and taken with meals
- Calming product to be taken during the day
- More of the same for stress and/or better night's sleep

Protocols by Conditions:

- Adrenal Protocol
- Diabetes II Protocol
- Autoimmune Protocol
- Pancreatitis Protocol
- Ulcerative Colitis Protocol
- Crohn's Disease Protocol
- Hepatitis Protocol
- Scleroderma Protocol
- Osteoporosis Protocol
- Mononucleosis Protocol
- Multiple Sclerosis
- Fibrocystic Breast Disease

STAGE SEVEN

This final cellular disorder stage involves tissue growth of a morbid nature. Poor circulation and general degeneration of the body is a result from the prior stages continued abuse. Poor eating habits, drugs that weaken the immune system, smoking, and unresolved stress upset the internal balance. The body's defense system breaks down as described above. The previous conditions of stages one to six have seriously compromised the body's ability to synthesize the needed metabolites, including metabolic enzymes and healthy cells.

It is this stage in which the cells can no longer adequately renew themselves. Tumors and other types of growths are encouraged to grow. Invasion of tumor cells into local tissue and their spread into distant organs underlies the phenomenon of metastasis (spreading of cancer). Metastasis is associated with 90 percent of cancer deaths.

There are over 150 different types of cancer, and they are a result of physical, nutritional, chemical and/or genetic mechanisms interfering with the normal function of the body's cells. As cells suffer the kind of progressive damage as seen in stages One through Six, they rob the other cells of nutrients, resulting in cellular "asphyxiation."

Additionally, cancer cells may be covered with a protein coat that help them be disguised and appear as normal cells ("self") thus helping them to evade the immune system. Damaged or abnormal cells are now left alone to coat themselves in glue-like fibers about 15 times the thickness of normal cells. They hide under this protective glue-like coating so that they cannot be recognized. These sticky cells wander around looking for a place to adhere so that they can build more fibrin and multiply, forming a tumor. The fiber around the cancer cell is made up of protein. Cancer cells are clever and have a "trademark" or cell markers. Even when the cell is destroyed, the trademark can get left behind. They are so smart that they can even leave a false trail so they can be undisturbed and can form new markers elsewhere. As more and more cancer cells with specific antigens invade the body, they overwhelm the immune system.

The body requires more systemic proteolytic enzymes for this protein fibrin. Digestive enzyme supplements will help in meeting the body's nutrient needs, especially in cases of cancer where metabolic needs are increased. Additionally, various studies have shown that proteases ingested orally help regulate cytokines in inflammation and play a helpful role in some forms of cancer.

Oncologists recognize that environmental, heredity, and biological factors play an important role in the development of cancer. Environmental causes are believed to account for at least 50 percent of many cancers. The AMA and Cancer Institutes of America have cited the results of poor digestive conditions are responsible for as high as 80 percent of many cancers.

IN CONCLUSION

Disease is not "bound to happen" and can be overcome if there is a willingness to eliminate all of the aforementioned abuses and maintain a disciplined adherence to a diet of life-giving foods.

The effect on the conditions by such a regime (digestive enzyme formulations, supplements, proper foods, and permanent life-changing habits) depends largely upon the extent of degeneration of affected vital organs.

If sufficient life-energy remains, the chance for rejuvenation is great. This is an example of the energy power within every human body. Remember that all symptoms mentioned are nothing more than the body's effort to return to balance.

Recommendations:

Ultimately, the prevention of cancer depends upon knowledge of each person's risk factors for the development of cancer, and that person's decision to avoid, whenever possible, those habits and practices that predispose that disease. If what the patients are doing is not working for them, then there must be a change—a possible 18-month program dependent on compliance.

Supplemental Recommendations:

- Enough supplemental digestive enzymes taken with meals
- At least 12 capsules of supplemental systemic protease enzymes if the formula contains at least 400 thousand HUT blended protease per capsule (take 3 capsules between meals 4 times a day)
- Healthy probiotics with meals and whatever the health professional determines is needed in addition to the base products

Eat only organic free from GMO foods, drink adequate pure water, and work on forgiveness and a positive outlook on your life.

NOTE: See Renewal Program

Chapter 12

Revitalize Your Energy Level

TAPPING YOUR LIFE FORCE

Are you happy with your energy level? If your answer is "no," you are not alone. Stress caused by career pressures, financial concerns, and relationship tensions can take a major toll on our bodies. This is particularly true for the endocrine and immune systems. These systems sense negative changes in our environment and send a corresponding message to the brain. If these two systems are already weakened by enzyme deficiency, the whole body can feel rundown and lethargic. As we age, the ability to produce sufficient amounts of digestive enzymes decreases. The lack of enzymes results in indigestion and/or malabsorption problems that can interfere with your sympathetic nervous system, hormones, and your brain.

What is the sympathetic nervous system? This part of our nervous system is responsible for crisis intervention. As an immediate response to danger or other traumatic challenges, the sympathetic nervous system puts body processes into high gear. It stimulates secretions from the endocrine glands. It pumps adrenaline into the system, while the adrenal glands themselves are releasing elevated levels of epinephrine into the bloodstream. The blood vessels constrict and sweating will begin in an effort to keep the body cool while under stress. All this working together is what gives the body its ability to flee or fight. The cost for this extra energy is the slowdown of the heart, lung action, and digestion. This is simply another example of the extraordinary functions our bodies are capable of performing.

If you have been told you have a thyroid problem or you are in adrenal fatigue, then this chapter is for you. To better understand how you got here, let's first understand the system both of these glands belong to.

WHAT IS THE ENDOCRINE SYSTEM?

Although we rarely think about them, the glands of the endocrine system and the hormones they release influence almost every cell, organ, and function of our bodies. We really do not tend to think of our other systems such as digestive or nervous systems unless we have a problem. The endocrine system is instrumental in regulating mood, growth and development, tissue function, and metabolism, as well as sexual function and reproductive processes.

In general, the endocrine system is in charge of body processes that happen slowly, such as cell growth. Digestive system gets the nutrients to the cell for its life, but faster processes like breathing and body movement are controlled by the nervous system. But even though the nervous system, digestive system, and endocrine system are separate systems, they often work together to help the body function properly.

The foundations of the endocrine system are the hormones and glands. As the body's chemical messengers, hormones transfer information via the enzymes from one set of cells to another. Although many different hormones circulate throughout the bloodstream, each one affects only the cells that are genetically programmed to receive and respond to its message. Hormone levels can be influenced by factors such as stress, infection, diet, and changes in the balance of fluid and minerals in blood.

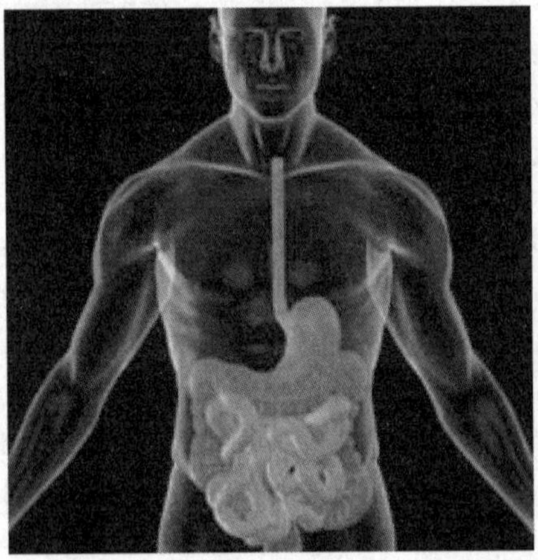

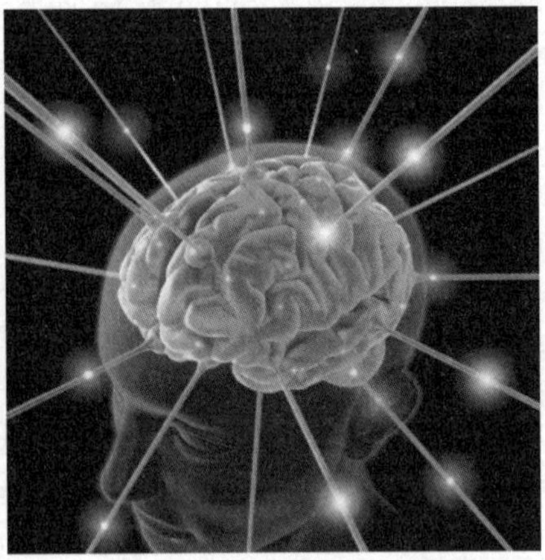

Endocrine Glands: A gland is a group of cells that produces and secretes, or gives off, chemicals. A gland selects and removes materials from the blood, processes them, and secretes the finished chemical product for use somewhere in the body. Some types of glands release their secretions in specific areas. For instance, exocrine glands, such as the sweat and salivary glands, release secretions in the skin or inside of the mouth. Endocrine glands, on the other hand, release more than 20 major hormones directly into the bloodstream where they can be transported to cells in other parts of the body.

Once a hormone is secreted, it travels from the endocrine gland through the bloodstream to target cells designed to receive its message. Along the way to the target cells, special proteins (enzymes) bind to some of the hormones. The special proteins act as carriers that control the amount of hormone that is available to interact with and affect the target cells.

For example, if the thyroid gland, which is in charge of your metabolism, has secreted adequate amounts of its hormone (thyroxin) into the blood, the pituitary gland must sense the level of thyroxin in the bloodstream and adjusts its release of TSH (stimulating hormone) to the thyroid. This is why when you have your thyroid blood levels taken they look at the TSH, T4, and T3. They are looking to see if your pituitary is releasing sufficient hormones in a normal range in order to stimulate your thyroid into producing sufficient thyroxin and if the thyroxin is being used correctly.

When things go wrong: Too much or too little of any hormone can be harmful to the body. Many clients have come to my office with conditions of fatigue and an overall feeling of un-wellness. After the usual interviews and tests and a close look at their medical histories, I recommend a diet to fit their biochemical type and a regimen of supplemental enzymes for them. The supplemental enzymes assist to rebuild the organs and tissues and strengthen all their processes to keep their bodies strong, refreshed, and balanced. After a few weeks have passed, I ask the key question: "Do you feel good?" If the answer is "yes," I know the enzymes are doing their job. If they say they still are not up to the energy they used to enjoy, I then add to the enzyme and glandular formulations to feed and fortify their endocrine system. When we reach the goal set by the client, we begin a reduction in the number of daily supplements, as long as good health and equilibrium remain stable.

Adrenal insufficiency. This condition is characterized by decreased function of the adrenal cortex and the consequent underproduction of adrenal corticosteroid hormones. The symptoms of adrenal insufficiency may include weakness, fatigue, abdominal pain, nausea, dehydration, and skin changes. Medical doctors treat adrenal insufficiency by giving replacement corticosteroid hormones. Here are natural ways to fortify the adrenal and that is in supporting the adrenal with its own glandular and the nutrients that particular gland requires. We have seen wonderful changes in their energy and frustration levels.

Hyperthyroidism. Hyperthyroidism is a condition in which the levels of thyroid hormones in the blood are excessively high. Symptoms may include weight loss, nervousness, tremors, excessive sweating, increased heart rate and blood pressure, protruding eyes, and a swelling in the neck from an enlarged thyroid gland (goiter). I have worked with this situation by bringing balance to the system with protease enzymes. Thyroxin is a protein hormone and many times taking the protease in the supplemental digestive formulas, along with the protease enzymes first thing in the AM and before bed, assists in balancing.

Hypothyroidism. Hypothyroidism is when the levels of thyroid hormones in the blood are abnormally low. Thyroid hormone deficiency slows body processes and may lead to fatigue, a slow heart rate, dry skin, weight gain, constipation, and, in kids, slowing of growth and delayed puberty. This is very common amongst the Americans. I believe it is so for several reasons. One is the removal of natural iodine in our food sources, genetically modified organisms GMO. The genetic proteins in our foods create confusion and cannot be absorbed creating a toxic overload. It makes logical sense to realize some of the problems are due to improper digestion of proteins. However, this is a simpler problem when you treat with thyroxin. I personally appreciate Armour Thyroid in place of the other medicines, which are just individual T4 or T3 when Armour thyroid contains T3, T4, and T7.

Type I Diabetes. When the pancreas fails to produce enough insulin, Type I Diabetes (previously known as juvenile diabetes) occurs. Symptoms include excessive thirst, hunger, urination, and weight loss. In children and teens, the condition is usually an autoimmune disorder in which specific immune system cells and antibodies produced by the immune system attack and destroy the cells of the pancreas that produce insulin.

Type I Diabetes can cause long-term complications, including kidney problems, nerve damage, blindness, and early coronary heart disease and stroke. To control their blood sugar levels and reduce the risk of developing diabetes complications, kids need regular injections of insulin. The side effects of insulin cause loss of digits. However, supporting the pancreas with supplemental digestive enzymes with meals and the protease between meals has worked for those that suffer with this condition.

Type II Diabetes. Unlike Type I Diabetes, in which the body can't produce normal amounts of insulin, in Type II Diabetes the body is unable to respond to insulin normally. Children and teens with this condition tend to be overweight, and it is believed that excess body fat plays a role in the insulin resistance that characterizes the disease. In fact, the rising prevalence of this type of diabetes in kids has paralleled the dramatically increasing rates of obesity among kids in recent years.

This is a condition that is driven by the foods we chose to eat including GMOs. We have had wonderful success with these people from the child through adult... Eating the proper genetic diet, taking supplemental digestive enzymes with meals,

Proteases between meals, and probiotics at bedtime. Since they can take their blood-glucose levels, they have a validation on the change of diet and enzymes.

INSOMNIA

Scientific research shows that those suffering from sleep deprivation or insomnia has some specific symptoms that are not experienced by normal sleepers. These are higher rectal temperatures, higher skin resistance, more constricting of the blood vessels per minute, and more body movements per hour. These characteristics are fine and are advantages in many different arenas in the workplace, but they are not conducive to good sleep.

The causes of insomnia may be physical or psychological or both. During sleep the metabolic rate should decrease approximately 10 percent below daytime levels. This drop is due to muscle relaxation and reduced activity of the sympathetic nervous system. The less relaxed your muscles are, the greater your metabolic rate. Any emotional strain can cause increased muscle tension with a corresponding upswing in metabolic rate. Personal problems and their attendant emotional stress, or other anxieties, can create a domino effect. The less we sleep, the more our bodies are susceptible to illness. Added to this we have a new anxiety to worry about—our inability to sleep. Insomnia can adversely affect not only our personal lives and our ability to do our work, but also our bodies' healing capabilities and energy levels.

Changing eating and sleeping habits easily solves some of the physical causes of insomnia. Caffeine drinks like coffee, tea, and cola speed up the metabolism, making it more difficult to sleep. Sugars have the same effect. Sometimes a softer or firmer mattress and pillows can allow for a more restful night's sleep. Avoiding heavy meals just before bed may also reduce the possibility of insomnia. If you have fibromyalgia, one type of dysfunctional sleep is called the alpha-delta sleep anomaly. As soon as people with FM reach the deep-level sleep, alpha brain waves invade and jolt them back to shallow sleep. Not only are they denied refreshing sleep, but the delta level is when the body does its repair work, chemical replenishment, and the making, as well as use of, the growth hormone.

If you have made these adjustments to no avail, I suggest supplemental plant-based enzyme supplementation. This supports your nervous system in general, but now we want to target the sympathetic nervous system. Remember, this is the part of the nervous system that creates increases in energy. The cost for this is the inability to relax into a restful rather than a restless state. Insomnia is another imbalance that has far-reaching effects. When we do not get a proper amount of sleep for our bodies, they cannot heal themselves. One of the reasons why the elderly often cannot sleep well is their bodies are becoming more and more metabolic enzyme deficient. Those over 50 do well with an addition of melatonin. Start with a low dose and work up to see which milligram is needed specifically for your need. You can find them anywhere from 1 mg up to 10 mg tablet or capsule. Those over 65 tend to take 30 mg time-released before bed.

CHRONIC FATIGUE SYNDROME

Chronic Fatigue Syndrome, or CFS, has been referred to as chronic Epstein-Barr virus, chronic mononucleosis, and Icelandic Disease, to name a few. Symptoms include fatigue, nausea, vomiting, abdominal cramping, muscle pain, joint aches, and lack of concentration. Millions of people suffer from one or more of these symptoms. Reports have indicated that more than 5 million persons in the United States have CFS. CFS cannot be diagnosed by standard tests, like urinalysis or blood work. Some medical personnel still will not acknowledge that it even exists, yet they are unable to explain the fatigue or illness that many people describe. Countless books have been written about Chronic Fatigue Syndrome. In every one of them, there is no shortage of radical diets to follow, herb mixtures, nutrients, and support groups.

CASE HISTORY

I have before me many charts with many similarities. However, Chronic Fatigue Syndrome manifests itself quite uniquely with each case that is documented. Four years ago, one of my clients came into my office with CFS symptoms. Here is her description of how she felt in her own words: *"I haven't felt well for the last eight months. I was okay for about a year before this, but now I am not able to hold down a regular job. My eyes feel tight and burn, and when they come into contact with water they sting. I have pressure in the head area, and I can't seem to think or function. My throat swells and feels like it is going to close sometimes. I have constant sore throats, and my lymph glands swell in my throat and underarms. My underarms sting when I perspire. Hives are brought on by heat or when I scratch myself. I tend to run fevers. My joints and muscles ache very badly at moments. I have trouble sleeping and wake up tired. I have pains in my chest, in fact when I get up, my right side feels like it is in a knot or swollen. I have a swelling in the liver and gallbladder area and sometimes you can even see it down at the bottom of my ribs. My feet ache most of the time and my hands go numb. I get chilled easily. I go from constipation to diarrhea. It is very easy for me to get short of breath. I have had kidney and bladder infections off and on. I experience PMS and cramps whether I am in my period or not. I have nausea, depression, and ringing in my ears."* She was frightened and discouraged. Various tests were performed that clearly showed her to be a textbook case. Realizing she had CFS, however, did nothing to help her recover. She tried every treatment known, but they made no difference.

Did she have CFS? A medical doctor had not diagnosed it, but she certainly had the symptoms. I promised her I would not lie to her and told her if she took supplemental enzymes she wouldn't recover immediately. However, if she would follow my suggestions and begin taking plant-based enzymes, I felt certain she would be back on the long road to better health. How would she know this? She would feel the difference in a few days, especially with the nausea. I gave her high potency digestive enzymes with her meals. She was on 330,000 units of protease five times a day, including between meals. Within the first 21 days she felt a marked improvement in controlling her headaches, nausea, vomiting, sore throat, muscle pains, and joint aches. The second 21-day period, she was working more hours per week at her job, and her diarrhea and constipation problems became balanced. Her chest pains disappeared and the swelling in her lymph nodes had noticeably reduced. Within nine weeks she was working full-time again. Up to this day, she is doing very well and living a full life. She cannot eat any junk food or drink alcohol without suffering ill effects, but she has gained control of her life. I treated her case over four years ago, and this young woman still uses enzymes and stays well.

On Thursday, July 17, 1997, Dr. Robert Suhadolnik and his research team at Temple University School of Medicine, Philadelphia, PA, reported that studies of patients with Chronic Fatigue Syndrome have led to the identification of a new human enzyme.

This new enzyme has lower molecular weight than the normal enzyme found in the viral pathway in which this protein is active and may explain common observations in patients with CFS. CFS patients have an inability to control common viruses and an inability to maintain cellular energy. According to Dr. Suhadolnik, the viral pathway known as the 2-5A Synthetase/RNaseL antiviral pathway may control both processes. He further stated, "This new enzyme in CFS may not function as well as the normal RNaseL found in healthy people. It may explain why CFS patients' bodies have a hard time maintaining the energy necessary for cellular growth."

As with any autoimmune disorder, dysfunction, or imbalance, I give the same regimen of supplemental enzymes, supported by a high dosage of protease. I believe in feeding and fortifying the endocrine and nervous systems while naturally detoxifying the body. With supplemental enzymes, all these things are possible. The endocrine system (glands that control all hormonal secretions), the nervous system, and the immune system must be addressed. Because they all function on enzymatic action, I know of no better way to support them other than through the use of enzyme supplements. Plant-based protease has a wide range of proteolytic activity. This means the body uses it where and when necessary.

HOW TO BOOST YOUR BRAIN ACTIVITY

Fatigue can be mild in some clients and yet incapacitating in others. The fatigue has often been described as "brain fatigue" in which clients are totally drained of energy. Remember the digestive system and the brain work together. Sometimes the patients are too tired to remember, let alone function at the moment. They tell me their brains are not functioning. Healthy brain activity requires healthy nerves, a powerful endocrine system, and a steady supply of oxygen and glucose. These requirements depend on a properly functioning digestive system. As we age, our bodies produce fewer hormones and chemicals critical for memory function. While memory loss in the elderly can be attributed to other sources, proper enzyme supplementation can help to fortify and restore the efficient operation of major organs. Insufficient exercise and inappropriate combinations of medication do cause memory loss in some users as a side effect. However, maintaining a proper balance of enzymes in our bodies can renew production of memory-enhancing substances. The results can be very impressive. Memory loss can be significantly reduced, and often halted altogether. The big lesson here is that it is much easier to prevent age-related memory loss than it is to restore it.

MYOFASCIA / CHRONIC FATIGUE / FIBROMYALGIA

Myofascia is a thin, almost translucent film that wraps around muscle tissue. It is the tissue that holds all the other parts of the body together. It gives you shape and supports all of the body's musculature. You can see myofascia if you cut up a fresh chicken. It is the thin, sticky, somewhat filmy material that wraps around the muscle tissue. It wraps around muscle fibers, bundles of fibers, and the muscles themselves, and then goes on to form tendons and ligaments. For people with fibromyalgia syndrome (FMS) and/or myofascial pain syndrome (MPS), the myofascia takes on a new importance. Tightening and thickening of the myofascia occurs in many cases of FMS and/or MPS. If both of these conditions are present, this tightening causes more than double the trouble. When the myofascial tissues become thickened and lose their elasticity, the neurotransmitter's ability to send and receive messages between the mind and body is damaged, and the communication between the mind and body is disrupted. Myofascia, then, may well be the key to what is wrong with FMS/MPS people. In myofascia, there is a material called ground substance. This material can exist in a solid, semisolid, or fluid state. When ground substance changes from a liquid to a gel, the myofascia tightens, and it is difficult to get it to reverse to a liquid state again without intervention.

MYOFASCIAL TRIGGER POINTS

Trigger Points (TrPs) are found as extremely sore points occurring in ropy bands throughout the body. They can also be felt as painful lumps of hardened fascia. The bands are often easier to feel along the arms and legs. If you stretch your muscle about 2/3 of the way out, you might be able to feel them. Sometimes the muscles get so tight that you can't feel the lumps, or even the tight bands. Your muscle feels like "hardened concrete." TrPs can occur in the myofascia, skin, ligaments, bone lining, and other tissues. They can be caused by a surgical incision, as is often the case with abdominal surgery. You have probably never heard of TrPs, yet they are quite common. Each specific TrP on the body has a referred pain or other symptom pattern that is carefully documented in the Trigger Point Manuals.

The first time I opened the Trigger Point Manuals (*Myofascial Pain and Dysfunction: The Trigger Point Manual, Vol. I & II* by Travell M.D. and David Simmons M.D.), I was dumbfounded. After being told for so many years by medical experts that the pain patterns I described did not and could not exist, seeing them illustrated in a medical text brought a flood of emotions. I felt so relieved and cried. I felt validated. Then, as the truth started to hit home, I started to get angry. Why didn't these "experts" have knowledge of Travell and Simmons' work? Why hadn't I learned about these texts in medical school? Most specific pains commonly attributed to FMS are actually from trigger points. TrPs seem to form throughout life as a response to many things that happen to our bodies. Overuse, repetitive motion trauma, bruises, strains, joint problems, etc. Pain creates a neuromuscular response, and the muscle around the pain site tightens, "guarding" the hurt area.

When muscles are in a state of sustained tension, they are working, even if you are not. A working muscle needs more nutrition and oxygen, and produces more waste, than a muscle at rest. This creates an area in the myofascia starved for food and oxygen, and loaded with toxic waste—a trigger point.

Dr. Janet Travell, in her autobiography, *Office Hours Day and Night*, explains how dizziness, ringing of the ears, loss of balance, and other symptoms can all be caused by TrPs in the side of the neck, in the muscle group called the sternocleidomastoid (SCM) complex. This muscle has many functions, one of which is to hold your head up. Receptors in the SCM complex transmit nerve impulses; inform the brain of the position of the head and body in the surrounding space. With TrPs, the receptors lie. What they tell the brain is not what the eyes tell the brain.

Developing secondary and satellite TrPs can give the false impression that the MPS is a condition that will steadily worsen with time—that it is progressive. MPS is not progressive. With the proper intervention, these trigger points can be broken up and eliminated.

FMS is, among other things, a systematic neurotransmitter deregulation, with many biochemical causes. There are other problems as well, but they are all systematic in nature, such as the alpha-delta sleep anomaly. Myofascial Pain Syndrome, however, is a neuromuscular condition. MPS happens because of mechanical failures—the mechanics of physics, not biochemistry. Due to the nature of trigger points, some of the symptoms may seem to be systemic, but they are not. Initiating events, such as repetitive motion injury, trauma, and illness, can start a cascade of TrPs. The protease that I have blended has shown to assist with this and inflammation.

FMS/MPS COMPLEX

People with the FMS/MPS Complex face more than just two sets of symptoms. Today, researchers are realizing that FMS and MPS not only occur together, but also reinforce each other. Therefore, physical therapy and all other forms of treatment must proceed carefully. Any treatment regimen will be more complicated and less successful than if the patient had only one of the two conditions. Only 20 percent of FMS cases have a known triggering event that initiates the first obvious "flare." During a flare, current symptoms become more intense, and new symptoms frequently develop. In FMS/MPS, a chronic pain condition exists, with many different symptoms. The trigger points of MPS are all magnified. The body's requirement for protease and lipase plant-based enzymes is greatly intensified. The necessity for supplemental enzyme therapy is essential for restoration. Systemic Protease enzymes taken between meals prevent chronic inflammation. I suggest taking these supplements often during the day.

CONCLUSION

Because this chapter is about energy I thought we should spend some time talking about how energy is produced. Without going into a great deal of biochemistry, I am going to make it a simple step-by-step picture. It takes a huge energy investment on the body's digestive system to make ATP (cellular energy). How our food is used to synthesize ATP is one of the great discoveries of modern biology because it comes from the food we digest.

- Our cells contain mitochondria—the tiny bodies where our ATP is produced.
- Mitochondria consist of two sacks made of membrane.
- The inner sack is ruffled or rumpled as to not be smooth as the outer sack.
- Sugar or glucose from food is fast energy, but our fat foods contain much more energy than glucose.

- They both can be found in between the ruffled and smooth sack in the mitochondria.
- In this area they are disassembled in a way to release their chemical bond.
- This energy imbeds the membrane, which push hydrogen ions into the ruffled inter-membrane sack as if it were a balloon.
- It is like blowing up a balloon and inserting it into inner membrane since this is where oxygen plays a role
- Oxygen has a powerful attraction for electrons.
- Think of the electrons like a stream of water and what oxygen does to the water in the stream by lowering it, allowing it to fit.
- Oxygen does this same thing to the electrons when they combine.
- If the oxygen was not involved, the mitochondria still could make around two ATP from the food source. But with the use of oxygen, they can produce around 36 ATPs from each energy molecule.
- Oxygen's powerful pull on electrons allows for it to push in hydrogen ions.
- The inner ruffled membrane is full of enzymes called ATP synthase
- Synthase enzymes create a hole through which the hydrogen ions can escape giving enough energy to create the bonds of ATP, and this is how our ATP battery is continually recharged.
- But now get this amazing thing—the leftover carbon atoms link with oxygen and leave the mitochondria by going into the blood stream where they are taken to the lungs for you to exhale.
- Oxygen in; waste out.

It is obvious to me when you do not eat healthy, or even if you do but cannot properly digest your food, you will be fatigued.

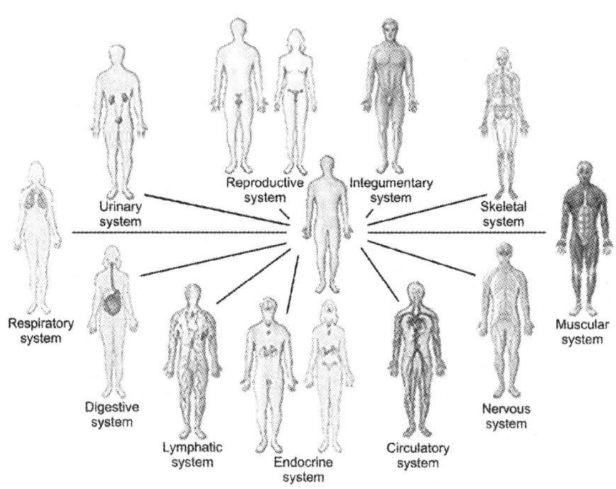

Chapter **13**

Pamper Your Sexuality

REVITALIZING YOUR SEXUAL HORMONES

Whenever a medical description is given of something as complex as a part of the human body, something gets lost in translation. The last thing I want to lose is the interest and attention of my readers! In short, your endocrine system is a family of glands that provide hormones for balance in the body. The major members of this gland family are the thyroid, parathyroid, pituitary, adrenals, the alpha and beta cells of the pancreas, and the gonads. The gonads are the sexual glands; testes in the male and ovaries in the female. Your endocrine system is one of only two major control systems in the body. The other one is the nervous system. They are very closely interrelated.

So what do glands do? Glands secrete hormones into your circulatory system, each of which is intended for a specific site within the body. These hormones control the tissues or other glands they reach by regulating the rates of chemical reactions inside the cells. Hormones have a profound effect on important functions such as growth, reproduction and the elimination of toxins. These chemical reactions must be precisely orchestrated so the targeted glands or tissues perform their tasks at the exact level of activity. If a healthy medium is not preserved, the originating gland or the target gland can be damaged. Some of the major illnesses that plague us arise when too few or too many hormones are released. We covered a few of them in Chapter 12. Now we will delve into the subject of hormones most people know about—Sex Hormones.

An example of this hormonal imbalance is menopause. When this stage of a woman's life arrives, the ovaries cease to produce estrogen. From that point on, she must depend on the adrenals to take up the production for her. Another situation could be when a person is unable to maintain a balance of calcium in his system. The thyroid, along with the rate of metabolism, regulates calcium levels. If the thyroid has been undermined, our ability to control our weight and our sleep patterns is adversely affected. When any of these situations take place, we are said to be suffering from a hormonal imbalance.

HORMONE IMBALANCE

A hormone is a substance formed in one gland and carried in the bloodstream to another gland or tissue where it serves a specific purpose. Although the total number of hormones the body produces is unknown, we do know that each hormone has its own unique chemical composition. Each gland of the endocrine system manufactures several different hormones. The adrenal gland alone produces more than 25 varieties of hormones. Growth, reproduction, sexual attributes, and personality traits are all dependent on hormones. Insulin is a well-known protein hormone that regulates carbohydrate metabolism. The beta glands in the pancreas produce it. Dr. William Regelson and Carol Colman did such a wonderful job describing the needs of hormone balance that I won't discuss into great detail in this book. I suggest reading *The Super Hormone Promise* (Simon & Schuster). In it, Dr. Regelson provides complete and comprehensive information about each of the super hormones, including up-to-the-last minute research on melatonin, DHEA, and pregnenolone.

If we want our bodies to function efficiently, our hormones must be in correct balance. Hormonal imbalances can cause problems ranging from lethargy to excitability. We now know that any significant imbalance in the kind and number of hormones generated must be corrected if we want our mind and bodies to be in a good state of health. I co-authored a book on menopause with a witty friend of mine which we named *The M Club*. For more information you might want to read that book. It was fun for me co-authoring with Wendy. She is one delightful lady and is known for designing clothes for the Barbie Doll. That will give you an idea what she looks like. However, like us normal gals, she is in menopause.

PREMENSTRUAL SYNDROME

In some cultures, the female cycle is considered an important time for women. It symbolizes a woman's power to create life. However, if you are a woman who suffers from Premenstrual Syndrome (PMS), you may not feel quite so powerful. While PMS manifests itself differently in different individuals, the most common physical symptoms are headaches, breast tenderness, weight gain, and sugar cravings. Some of the psychological effects include mood swings, depression, irritability, fatigue, and tension. There have been 150 symptoms of PMS reported. Many causes have been proposed for it: Estrogen compared to a progesterone imbalance, how the body metabolizes glucose, a deficiency of the brain chemical serotonin, hypoglycemia, and candida. Women who are most likely to develop PMS are those who suffer from sugar imbalance and intolerance.

I suggest many different preventive methods for dealing with PMS. Women suffering from PMS should avoid caffeine, excessive salt, alcohol, and smoking. Abstention from these toxins should always be observed, not just before or during the menstrual period. Increasing your intake of complex carbohydrates, proteins, and exercise helps considerably in the management of stress due to PMS. A good 30-minute walk every day does wonders for reducing susceptibility. Supplemental enzymes can be used as prevention for PMS. I advise women to increase their protease dosage 10 days before their period and make some diet changes as well. Protease should be taken in the mornings, evenings, and mid-afternoons. Protease will assist with controlling your inflammation and bloating during this time. A digestive formulation high in lipase and protease will help sugar cravings to subside.

One of the questions appearing on my health questionnaire asks if you have suffered, or do you have PMS. Almost all women answer "yes" to this question. PMS is regarded as a disorder or symptom that makes you feel unwell during the time of menses. Is there a way we can prevent this before we ever experience the first symptom? The answer is "yes" and the preventatives are enzymes. I think it is wonderful that education and information about enzymes is becoming much more widespread than it was several years ago. Since 1986 I have seen young parents starting their children on an enzyme program at early ages. Young girls who have been on enzymes have a significantly lesser occurrence of PMS than others. Even after symptoms are observed, something can be done to alleviate the chaos caused in the body from PMS.

CASE HISTORY

A 16-year-old girl came to see me. About two weeks of her month are fairly normal. But the other two are full of mood swings, cramps, and a good case of the "uglies," as she puts it. Her mother had taken her to several OB/GYN doctors and nothing worked except heavy doses of prescription drugs. The mother did not want her daughter to have to endure her teenage years in a drugged stupor, although her father thought that might be a very good idea! I suggested the basic regimen of enzymes, but reminded the girl it was her responsibility to follow the directions. I asked her to make another appointment with me after she had two more periods, during which time she would be using the enzymes.

She reported that her first period under the enzyme program seemed easier. Instead of her usual bloating and depression, her period started before she even realized it. She was sure that "It was all in my head." With the second cycle there were no cramps, bloating, or depression. I modified her enzyme dosage and explained to her that she would no longer have mood swings if she gave up soft drinks and candy bars. I told her to eat more protein foods. She called to cancel her appointment that had been scheduled right after her third period. She said she did not need to come in, that all her symptoms were gone. By learning which foods triggered her anger and other symptoms, she has eliminated them from her diet. Coupled with an increase in her protease, she feels great.

Premenstrual symptoms are reality. Many women suffer from them. I encourage you to do what you can to relieve the symptoms. Often, the solution is to educate yourself and find out what works best for you. When you have a strong sugar craving, this is your body's way of telling you it needs nutrients or wants support. There is a big difference between this and how we mistakenly think our bodies need sugar. The more sugar you eat, the more the brain cries out for nutrients, and you think that means more sugar. Hence, the roller coaster ride never comes to an end. When you fortify your body and give it what it needs, the cravings disappear. Taking carbohydrate-splitting enzymes, the enzymes that break down all the carbs and sugars you crave and eat, will assist you in overcoming irresistible temptations. If you continue to support your system with enough carbohydrate-splitting enzymes, you will discover that even you—yes, you—can give up sugar. I recommend the dosage for protease to be 375,000 or higher units of activity taken at one time. For PMS, you might want to try a good carbohydrate digestive enzyme formula to dispel the yearning for sugars. Foods that break down to a fast sugar or glucose are usually starches and desserts. These are actually part of the reason for your inflammation and bloating.

MENOPAUSE

Menopause, or the "Change of Life," occurs when a woman's menstrual cycle wanes and gradually stops. Along with this, the ovaries stop functioning. This natural process is the result of the normal aging of the ovaries and occurs when they can no longer generate ovulation and estrogen production. While the first and most obvious sign of menopause is the change in menstrual flow, the gradual cessation of estrogen production causes many physiological changes. The fallopian tubes, uterus, cervix, and vagina all become smaller. The average American woman will experience pre-menopause between the ages of 47 to 51. Almost 75 percent of women will begin the peri or pre menopause in their 40s. In some instances, it can begin as early as 35 or start as late as 55. Menopause should be a late 50 to 60 complaint, and if you are suffering earlier then it is usually due to hormonal imbalance brought on by toxicity or poor digestion. What we eat influences our ability to continue the hormone production, such as properly breaking down fats encourages the steroid hormone production, and properly breaking down proteins assist the thyroid and other peptide-producing hormones.

Surprisingly to many women going through forced toxic menopause, when consuming supplemental digestive enzymes their period begins. They are quick to accuse me of making this take place but I always encourage them to do what is natural for their bodies rather than to age earlier than necessary.

The length of time it takes to complete menopause varies, but it usually lasts anywhere from six months to three years. Most women pass right through menopause with little discomfort. Only about 15 percent experience discomfort and distress. Occasionally during menopause, some existing physical ailments may become exaggerated. Hot flashes, one of the most common symptoms of menopause, are sensations of heat in the face and upper body. I have had many women come through the clinic suffering with premature menopause that goes on for too many years.

Too often chills follow the heat sweats. Some women feel just a few of these hot flashes over a period of time, while others can experience 10 to 20 per day. Those women who do suffer psychological reactions may experience fatigue, crying episodes, insomnia, an inability to concentrate or lapses in memory. More severe reactions may result in depression. At one time it was thought that the changes in the body's chemistry caused these reactions. Today, many physicians believe that chemical changes that bring on menopause simply trigger reactions to other events that occur at this time of life. We need to be aware that as we age we lose digestive enzymes along with the enzymes that produce DHEA. There is a lot of information available on DHEA, melatonin and the youth hormones but virtually nothing on the enzymes required for these hormones to work.

CASE HISTORY

Menopausal women who have used enzyme therapy report that their hot flashes and night sweats are things of the past. One 49-year-old woman was experiencing fatigue, hair loss, hot flashes, depression, and insomnia. Although she tried under-the-counter menopausal remedies, she found no relief from these serious symptoms. As soon as she began treating her entire body, especially her endocrine and nervous systems with enzyme therapy, her condition began to improve. Her hair was healthy, her depression and fatigue lifted, and she began to sleep at night, free of hot flashes.

In other cultures and in times past, a woman who gave up her blood (entered menopause) could at last hold in her own energy and power. Known as crones, they were regarded as the most powerful and wisest of women. Within a tribe, clan, or village, they were highly valued and revered. Nowadays, many women in our culture live for over 80 years. A full one-third of these women's lives are lived after menopause has come and gone. It should not be looked upon as a curse or an illness any more than menstrual periods. It is not an enemy.

SURGICAL MENOPAUSE

If a woman has her ovaries surgically removed, she experiences menopause immediately. This is because most of her natural estrogen production has been terminated. This menopause can be more traumatic because the body was not given time to gradually accept the loss of estrogen production. Enzyme therapy can make this process less emotionally disturbing by supporting the endocrine system. The enzymes aid in helping the body adjust to the estrogen loss. Eventually it will resume production of its own metabolic enzymes and call on the other hormonal organs to produce.

I know this to be a fact since I went through surgical menopause at the age of 28 and did not have to address hormone issues until I was age 60.

HORMONAL REPLACEMENT THERAPY (HRT)

Should you or shouldn't you? Hormonal Replacement Therapy, or HRT, involves taking synthetic estrogen when the ovaries no longer produce it. HRT is certainly not for all women. The decision to take it is very much an individual one. There have been many findings and recommendations published from all the research done on this controversial topic. Estrogen replacement was introduced in Germany in 1896 where ovarian extracts were used. Today, in our own age of chemicals, estrogen is commercially prepared. Synthetic estrogen is the most commonly used medication on today's market. In the 50s and 60s, estrogen therapy was touted as "feminine forever." During the 70s, some studies indicated that the use of synthetic estrogen had cancer-causing effects on the lining of the uterus. Then 1980 and the ensuing decade we were told if we added progesterone, the harmful side effects of HRT would be easier to control. In the 90s, we started questioning the use of chemicals, pills, patches, creams, injections, implants, and sublingual (under-the-tongue) therapies. Countless books on the subject denote a bewildering array of information. At the first glance, it would seem that estrogen replacement is the answer. However, each book I have read ended in doctors' cautioning it was not for everyone. No wonder there are so many confused women struggling with this decision that is critical to their health.

HARVARD NURSES STUDY

This was a well-publicized example of hormone replacement therapy and heart attack risks for postmenopausal women. In brief, the observational study gave misleading answers because the "treatment" and "control" groups differed systematically. In this ongoing investigation, begun in 1976, the researchers examined the impact of long-term HRT use in more than 60,000 nurses. They looked at length and continuity of hormone use and how this affected the women's death rates. They also studied women who used estrogen alone or in an estrogen/progesterone combination and adjusted their data to account for smoking, weight, exercise, and other lifestyle habits. Overall, the researchers found that the death rate among HRT users was 37 percent lower than that of women who had never taken hormones, primarily because the hormones appeared to protect women against heart disease. Indeed, the risk of dying of cardiovascular disease was 53 percent lower in the HRT group.

Then the evidence from the Women's Health Initiative, a randomized clinical trial from the 1990s, is that hormone replacement therapy increases the risk of heart attack in older women.

NIH: Do not use estrogen plus progestin therapy to prevent heart disease. The new findings show that it doesn't work. In fact, the therapy increases the chance of a heart attack or stroke. And it increases the risk of breast cancer and blood clots.

2012 NIH changed their mind saying the study was fundamentally flawed. The analysis found that all three studies failed to meet the majority of the criteria and therefore none of the studies was able to establish whether HRT increases the risk of breast cancer.

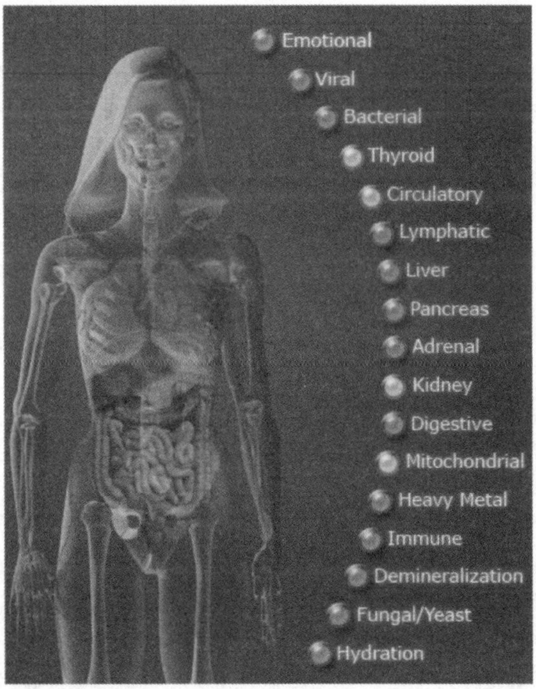

GOOD GRIEF...READY TO THROW IN THE TOWEL?

Current reports Indlcate that less than 20 percent of menopausal women choose hormonal replacement therapy. The decision about this treatment is highly personal, and depends on a woman's family history, personal habits, and the risk factor she finds the most tolerable. This is not a one-size-fits-all situation. In my work, the question arises: "Can the woman who is a longtime follower of natural health approaches skip HRT without damaging her health? Dr. Regelson describes the new "designer" estrogens that are being offered. The estrogen needs are different from woman to woman.

I personally choose to use natural ingredients (bio-identical) hormones delivered by enzymes, even though I had a hysterectomy at the age of 28. I have also experienced hormone pellets, which are put in just under the skin, and they are utilized by blood flow. It is a natural way to have the hormones delivered on need. Some hormones are taken orally which involve progesterone or pregnenolone and DHEA delivered by the enzyme lipase. I would never tell anyone what to do. This happens to be my personal choice, and it works for me. I am now in my 70s and feel very healthy and vibrant. Again, it must be a personal choice. I believe the important word here is "choice." What are your choices?

BHRT "Bio-Identical hormones" seems to mean different things to different individuals. Bio-identical hormones are hormones that have a compound composition that's identical to the hormones that are created by our bodies. The doctors that are offering these compounded therapies base them on your hormone panel results. Bio-Identical hormones have grown in popularity in recent times, partially due to movie star endorsements and partially in response to reviews of elevated health threats that may be posed by normal hormonal treatments.

Typically they are created from the different parts of plants, usually compounds obtained in soybeans or Mexican wild yams and they're chemically the same as human bodily hormones, to fit precisely the formulation that a woman's own body generates, so that they are recognized by her body to be a naturally occurring substance and thus can be used by the body in natural and non-intrusive manner.

When you compare bio-identical hormones to the pharmaceutically-created artificial hormone types, or pregnant horse urine, the studies show that very frequently the results obtained by each group are completely different. This along with the total distrust and frustration that many holistic practitioners feel towards the FDA has caused a pretty fiery debate on the safety of these bio identical hormones. So as one may have anticipated, the use of bio-identical hormone replacement therapy (BHRT) vs. prescription-based HRT drugs has prompted a large amount of consumer attention, in addition to hot debate.

A lot of women encounter estrogen dominance, a common condition in which a woman may have too much estrogen with very little, if any, progesterone to balance its effects within their bodies. There are three forms of estrogen created within the body: estriol, estrone, and estradiol. Progesterone is anabolic steroid hormone produced by the ovaries during the middle of the menstruation period. Progesterone is regarded as the most widely used bio-identical hormone, with more than 30 years of usage in the USA.

The human body is a great marvel. The endocrine glands secrete vital hormones, which control many bodily functions. Everything is designed to be perfectly synchronized when optimum health prevails. If hormone production is less than adequate, it is because the once reliable glandular systems are unbalanced and weak. One of the miracles of our natural design is the manner in which the body compensates for lost or damaged components. For example, when the ovaries have been surgically removed or cease to function because of menopause, other glands fulfill the need for estrogen. These glands release hormones that perform all the functions of estrogen except sustaining the menstrual cycle. These glands are also a part of the endocrine system.

This raises another question: Why do we need estrogen replacement, or why do we have PMS if other glands produce hormones that seem to replace estrogen? When the organs and systems of the body are in a depressed state, we cannot expect them to do everything it is programmed to do without some external support. This is why women often have to opt for BHRT. In fact, it is an enzyme called telomerase that assists in the making of the hormone that stops aging. If you are missing this enzyme, the whole hormonal cascade unwinds.

Our endocrine system is often referred to as the "body mind." This will give you a good feel for how vitally important it is. It virtually runs the systems of the body. The hypothalamus in the brain sends signals to the pituitary—the master gland. The pituitary is responsible for distributing this information to all other glands by hormones, moving in the bloodstream. This can be likened to a fine quality, state-of-the-art, high tech piece of electronic equipment. Because it is so fine-tuned, no electrical shorts can occur. However, if the endocrine system is not running at maximum efficiency, it malfunctions. It can no longer meet the demands of the body. This system runs on enzymatic action, as does the nervous system. When the glands are undernourished, it takes enzymes to deliver the nutrients from the food or vitamin and mineral supplements. Without enzymes, these nutrients cannot be assimilated.

I have counseled thousands of menopausal women. They all have many things in common. The one ailment we can eradicate completely is hot flashes and the attendant night sweats. These symptoms do not stop immediately; however with the enzyme therapy, combined with correct foods for an individual's biochemical type, it's only a matter of weeks before they dissipate. This usually takes 21 days. I have known some women who have experienced remarkable changes in only three days.

CASE HISTORIES

A 51-year-old woman came to me for nutritional advice. She did not mention that she was having severe hot flashes, because she believed everyone had them—they came with the territory. I helped her determine her biochemical type, and she proceeded with her enzyme therapy. I did not give her the extra enzyme mixture I normally give to menopausal women. I did not ask, and she did not volunteer any information. After three days, she called to ask if she was hallucinating. She was amazed that her hot flashes had drastically decreased. It is very rewarding for me to see these changes take place in my clients, especially when there are no expectations involved. Many women survive PMS and its rigors for the same reason. When the body begins to balance, it heals itself. When the glands are well-nourished, the body will not suffer from malfunction or malnutrition.

Another lady who came to see me was in the state of great anxiety. She was 49. Her face was breaking out, she was losing her hair, she would wake at two o'clock in the morning, unable to go back to sleep; she was exhausted. None of the menopausal aid products she obtained from the health food store had worked for her. She could not continue, her life was not working. Whatever she tried, relief would not come to her. I told her that she had to feed and fortify her body, and treat it with great love. Although she had taken the creams mixed with different herbs to increase progesterone, there had to be more things done to complete the balance. I knew her endocrine system had been badly undermined. When a woman enters menopause, she can no longer count on her ovaries for hormonal support. She must rely on her adrenal, her thyroid and the other glands of the endocrine system. This woman, my client, finally understood that she could not get by on over-the-counter quick fixes. She had to treat her body as an interdependent organism. When she began using the enzymes, she made tremendous progress in only 21 days.

There has been a common agreement between those that come to me for counseling and myself. We commit to a program for at least six weeks, but preferably nine weeks. The ideal time is nine weeks. The lady whose case I just reviewed for you had become so deficient, with a very weak immune system that I kept her on quite an intense dosage for four or five months. But what works for one does not work for all. The enzymes always work, but the time frame can vary greatly, depending on an individual's needs. Her need was greater than in the first woman's case. The first step is always to determine where you are in your own healing or enervation process. That way, you can decide how long you need to treat and feed yourself. To expect to turn your state of health around in only three days is unrealistic. I would encourage all women who are entering menopause to give themselves time to heal. Remember, educating yourself is the key; only then make choices that fit your lifestyle.

Remember...The enzymes always work, but the time frame can vary greatly, depending on an individual's needs.

Different biochemical types respond differently to estrogen therapy. The Type Four biochemical types, those who are underdeveloped or boyish, respond well to it. This is because their estrogen levels were low in the first place. The Type Three biochemical types, or overly developed women, however, do not respond as well. These women tend to have larger breasts and experience blood sugar problems. The Type Three already have high estrogen, as do the Type Two biochemical type. Both Type Three and Type Four seem to be irritated by estrogen replacement therapy. For these latter two types, I make sure they feed and fortify their entire endocrine system. I would never ask a client to stop taking estrogen if her personal physician had prescribed it for her.

Those women who do not do well with HRT have a connection with the way they are built (genetics) and with some of their food cravings. Some of the symptoms that may occur while on estrogen are fatigue, depression, moodiness, bloating, headaches, or irritable bowel movements. I suggest ways to support these problem areas so the client can make her own choice about whether or not she wants to continue with estrogen or try another therapy. One of these choices is wild yam cream with progesterone, which can be purchased from health food stores, some clinical nutritionists, or other health-care professionals. For a woman who wants to take the natural path, some suggestions are: Enzyme therapy, natural hormones, pregnenolone, DHEA and lipase, food vitamins and minerals from natural herbs, or glandular specific to the endocrine glands, a biochemical type food plan that specifically suits you, extra protein for insulin control, stress management, powerful thinking, attitude, relaxation, expressing your feelings and needs in an appropriate manner, living in the moment, laughter, visualizing yourself as you want to be, and exercise. Whew!

It needs to be noted that there is a sequential order in the hormonal balancing system. This order is as follows: Good insulin balance which in turn affects healthy DHEA balance, which in turn affects every hormone in the body. Enzymes directly affect this entire sequential order. The precursor to DHEA is the hormone pregnenolone, which ceases to be produced when enzyme production stops. This situation raises the age-old "chicken and egg" question: Do we age because our enzyme production stops or does enzyme production stop because we age? If you desire more information on menopause I co-authored "The M Club" where you can get more detailed information.

PROSTATE PROBLEMS

The American Cancer Society estimated in 2013 that 238,590 men would be diagnosed with prostate cancer and 29,720 would ultimately die of it. Researchers do not know what causes prostate cancer, although it occurs more frequently in older men, men with a family history of cancer, and Hispanic and African-American men. If detected early, prostate cancer can be treated with radiation, drugs, or surgery. From my own experience, I have observed that most men who have prostate problems enjoy fatty or salty foods, and may also have a sweet tooth. It is now 2014 and there have been many breakthroughs in Prostate Cancer and treatments.

Swollen prostates do not necessarily mean cancer. However, if swelling is involved, a medical doctor will closely monitor this patient to watch for signs of the onset of cancer. Men who are vegetarians tend to have less susceptibility to prostate cancer. If the prostate is swollen, painful and frequent urination is a symptom. After beginning enzyme therapy, this discomfort will dissipate. Doctors have found that men using this therapy experience reduced swelling in their prostates. I have them take concentrated dosages of protease and lipase enzymes. Protease in massive doses does cause frequent urination, but it relieves the pain caused by the swelling. As in the case of the woman who did not bother to mention her hot flashes, many of my male clients will mention, after the fact, how much better their prostates feel after regular enzyme therapy.

CASE HISTORY

A 55-year-old man with an enlarged prostate began enzyme therapy under my guidance. He added some necessary diet changes to his program as well. His doctor decided not to proceed with the scheduled surgery that had been planned. Instead, the man had begun eating raw foods like salads, fruits, and vegetables, and had cut back on his intake of spicy foods. He eliminated red meat from his diet but continued eating fowl, fish, and organic foods. He took high dosages of protease in the morning, midmorning, mid-afternoon, and evening. The swelling of his prostate went down along with the urinary discomfort. He is doing beautifully and has recommended that several of his friends with similar problems come to see me for nutritional counseling.

BALANCING AND STABILIZING YOUR HORMONES

Hormones are very powerful substances, and extremely small amounts are sufficient to accomplish the work for which they are intended. These chemical messengers are released into the bloodstream by endocrine glands. Their mission is to travel through the bloodstream and lymphatic systems as regulators of the physiological activities of cells or organs. When the hormones arrive at their destination, they act as stimulants for certain receptor cells. The ultimate goal is to create and maintain homeostasis, your internal equilibrium and a balanced body.

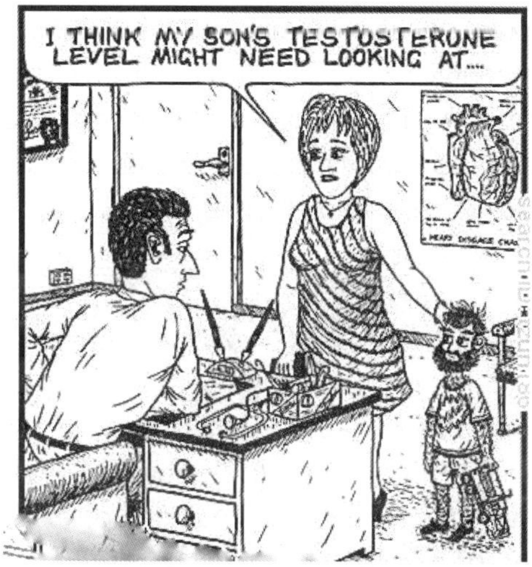
I THINK MY SON'S TESTOSTERONE LEVEL MIGHT NEED LOOKING AT....

There are specific hormones such as estrogen, testosterone, cortisone, and insulin that shows us beyond doubt how interrelated the endocrine system is with the rest of the body. These miracle substances have amazing powers, effecting dramatic changes in everything from pain control to the sex drive and mood swings. Imbalance can occur when certain tissues and glands become too active or too inactive because the hormone support released from a regulatory gland was either insufficient or excessive. To maintain a healthy body, you must be sure your glands are getting enough proteins. But that is not enough. These must be usable proteins. These proteins must be of a kind that will be metabolized into useful amino acids. The best way to obtain these proteins is through a proper diet and appropriate enzyme supplements so that the body can correctly digest and deliver these proteins. This is certainly where biochemical types become important. When you know your biochemical type, you can determine the best sources of protein for you to eat. The wrong proteins can interfere with the acid/alkaline balance necessary for good health.

It is not unusual for women to come in for counseling and tell me they have already experienced early menopause. I am very honest with them when I warn them, "Please understand that the body may be in a state of imbalance and when we begin to give it what it needs, like life-giving enzymes, it is normal for those in 'early menopause' to begin having periods again." This is met with a variety of responses.

CASE HISTORY

One young married woman who had not experienced regular periods for years came to my office. She had given up on becoming a mother; at the very least she wanted a healthier life. Several doctors she had seen throughout her married life told her she was unable to conceive. She had not felt well for a long time and wanted something to boost her energy level. Enzyme therapy proved to be exactly what she needed. Her periods started again and began to be regular. Within a few months she was pregnant! I did not promise her or give her hope that pregnancy would occur. I simply pointed out to her that I could advise her on body needs. When life-giving enzymes are taken, the body responds.

Major problems and illnesses can afflict us when our bodies get out of balance. Another way to state this is that certain glands and tissues become too active or too inactive. A healthy network is absolutely essential to good health. The purpose of this chapter is to make you aware that many of the hormonal imbalances that men and women suffer can be arrested, or better yet, prevented. We fear those things we do not understand. Spending time educating ourselves about preventatives is time well spent.

Two big warning signals are sent out in the form of prostrate swelling or painful urination. Another signal is ongoing fatigue and a feeling of being out of sync with the rest of the world. These warnings must be addressed, not ignored. This is what prevention is all about. We must learn to anticipate problems by stopping or blocking them. How do we do that? Simply by giving life back to our bodies with living foods and supplemental enzymes. Think about it. What makes the most sense? If every action, including hormonal action, is run by enzymatic activity, does it not make a great deal of sense to keep the body fortified with a continuous supply of supplemental enzymes?

Chapter 14

Forever Young with Skin Renewal

REAL REJUVENATION MUST COME FROM WITHIN; IT IS NOT A TOPICAL PROCESS

As we grow older, the body's ability to manufacture enzymes slackens. The enzyme content in the body tissues and fluids decreases with the natural aging process as well as with the onset of disease. Investigators at Michael Reese Hospital found that older people had less starch digesting enzymes (amylase) in their saliva than younger people.

Dr. Edward Howell has stated that the faster you use up your body's enzyme supply, the faster you will exhaust your enzyme reserve or enzyme potential. This depletes the body's limited enzyme capacity and he believed this is one of the paramount causes of aging and early death." In other words, forcing your body to produce enzymes for digestion limits its ability to manufacture the metabolic enzymes needed to build and repair the body. Supplementing your diet with enzymes not only aids digestion, but it also helps to build, repair, and rejuvenate the body, making the most of your enzyme potential.

We all feel pride when our skin is clear, smooth, and radiant. We cringe when it is dry, crusted, sallow, wrinkled, and lifeless. Products that offer skin renewal are like magnets for most of us. Oddly enough, enzymes are mostly ignored in this ongoing quest. However, they play a vital role in skin care and maintenance.

Enzymes are directly related to the health and appearance of our skin. They are the catalysts (increases the rate of chemical reactions without changing themselves) that work in healthy digestion, freeing the nutrients in our food that will form the building blocks for our glowing skin. Enzymes are the power source behind efficient circulation that will bring nutrients to the skin. Enzymes are responsible for reducing the unsightly signs of detoxification that come through our skin.

They slow the aging process that is evident in sagging and wrinkled skin. In this chapter, I will cover how enzymes hold the aging process at bay. You will learn how enzyme therapy will enhance your personal skin care.

FEEDING FROM WITHIN

The manufacturers of commercial beauty products are well aware of the American obsession with young-looking, healthy skin. They produce creams, lotions, gels, peels, pads, ointments, and masks for a wide assortment of skin needs and problems. The prestigious brands command as much as $100 an ounce for rejuvenating cream. The reality, however, is this: Real rejuvenation must come from within; it is not a topical process.

The nourishment it receives from the blood determines the health and appearance of your skin. The skin's under-layer, or dermis, is made up of collagen (protein). Collagen extracts the nutrients it requires from the blood. The outer layer of the skin, the epidermis, is not nourished from within. It continually dies and sloughs off, allowing the new skin cells of the dermis to rise to the surface. This creates an ongoing process of continuously renewing the skin that is fed from its deeper layers. Our skin is not just a few layers but 32 layers thick. That is why digestive enzymes play such a vital role in healthy skin upkeep. Enzymes are directed to the rich nutrients that must be available for skin nourishment.

DIGESTIVE ENZYMES

The skin needs to be fed with the nutrients from fats (fat-soluble vitamins), proteins, amino acids for the collagen and carbohydrates (water-soluble vitamins) in order to remain healthy and vibrant. If your digestive system has an enzyme deficit, these nutrients stay locked inside the foods you've eaten. They will not be broken down properly and will exit the body undigested. The skin becomes undernourished, weak and susceptible to problems.

DIGESTIVE ENZYME DEFICIENCIES

All of us should have plenty of naturally occurring nutrients in our diets. The digestive system calls its own enzymes to break down foods and unlock nutrients. Many believe raw foods contain their own supply of digestive enzymes (which they do) but humans do not use them for digestion. These types of enzymes are turned off or made dormant by our stomach acid. The condition of our skin may improve from the wonderful nutrients which are intact in the foods but not because of the raw food enzymes. I educated you in the chapter on enzymes on raw foods. There is nothing as full of nutrients as plant foods for our skin.

Our genetic programming, which happens in the womb, determines biochemical type and the result can cause us to have difficulty in the digestion of certain foods. Type One has trouble with most carbohydrates, even vegetables and fruit. Type Two does not properly break down fats or starch. Type Three cannot efficiently digest all protein. The Type Four encounters problems with dairy products and many carbohydrates.

When the body is unable to produce digestive enzymes for any of these reasons, you will surely see it in the appearance of the skin. A shortage of protease is especially noticeable in the skin. This is because the dermis feeds primarily on protein. Protease breaks down protein to make it readily available to the cells. Without enough protease, the skin can literally starve from the lack of its requirement for amino acids.

SEEING IS BELIEVING

A proper supply of supplemental plant-based digestive enzymes will improve the overall look and feel of your skin. If you are suffering from skin disorder, then I suggest taking a good source of protease systemic enzymes between meals. They are blended to work in the blood and can assist in ridding the body of toxins. The regenerative and healing power of enzymes will show up most dramatically in cases of visible skin disorders. A good example is acne, which is a problem with hormones and properly digesting fat. Adding lipase to the protease between meals will assist in this disorder.

I want to share with you a remarkable example of healing skin with enzymes. This is my own story. When I was a child, I had eczema virtually all over my body. It was especially severe in the creases of my arms and legs, eyes, and mouth. At times, the sores were so unsightly and painful that I had to stay home from school. Following doctor's orders, my parents would wrap me in cloths soaked in medication. I would lie in bed and cry, wearing my "mummy" prescription. My eczema was the weeping kind; if I scratched the sores, or if they cracked from dryness, they would weep and then spread. I cannot tell you how uncomfortable I was or how embarrassed I felt during these years of affliction.

As I grew, eczema episodes came less often and were less severe, but I was never completely free of its dry patches and scales. Whenever I was under stress, I would break out in the corners of my eyes, mouth and the creases of my arms. The outbreaks aggravated the stress response and the cycle of discomfort, embarrassment, and cancelled appointments would repeat themselves.

Later, I began to learn about the skin-healing effects of enzymes and was anxious to try them on myself. I began with a multi-digestive enzyme supplement and took these along with my three main meals. I also took high doses of protease between meals on an empty stomach. I have continued with this therapy to this very day and have never once had a recurrence of the eczema that plagued me for more than 35 years of my life. It was when I gave my body the proteases between meals for my cancer that I noticed my eczema went away and has no longer been a problem.

DETOXIFICATION IS IMPORTANT

Along with the kidneys, bowel, lungs, the body for detoxification uses the skin. Incomplete elimination of toxins through the kidneys takes place when we have trouble with urination or simply do not drink enough water. The same problem occurs in the bowel when we suffer constipation or lose our fluids by diarrhea. The lungs cannot do their part in detoxification if we smoke tobacco or breathe polluted air. What is left? Our skin then takes over the job. This is painfully brought to our attention in noticeable conditions like acne, eczema, psoriasis, pimples, blackheads, Lipoma, and for we women, cellulite.

FIGHTING OFF FREE RADICALS

In addition to the natural process of elimination, the body is in a continuous detoxification battle with free radicals. These invaders roam through our bodies on an endless search-and-destroy mission. The pollutants we breathe, the hormones and antibiotics we ingest in our meats, the pesticides we consume on our fruits and vegetables, the bacteria, fungi, and parasites to which we are exposed, are just a few of the toxins that must be eliminated from our systems.

There are no more powerful scavenger antioxidants than supplemental plant based protease enzymes. They grab on to the free radicals before they can do their damage. Think of them as a "Pac Man" because they actually look like them as they go in for toxins and then carry them away to be sent from the system. Any cellular debris left over after an attack is hauled away by these proteolytic molecules. These enzymes clean up free radical damage in cell membranes. They can actually enter the cell's control center and help repair devastation by free radicals to its DNA.

An ever-present supply of enzymes reduces future damage to the skin by toxins. Enzymes can even repair cells that are already impaired by free radicals. Enzymes are the only substances in the body that can rebuild injured cells by infusing them with oxygen and fortifying nutrients.

SIGNS OF DAMAGE

The effects of unchecked toxins on our skin can clearly be observed. Incomplete digestion and the adverse action of free radicals cause skin disorders in the majority of American adults. The remedy is supplemental multi-enzyme therapy. Major enzymes work together to address skin eruptions. Any sores, blemishes, lesions, or blisters on the skin are known as eruptions. Protease and lipase combine digestive and detoxifying action to manage the following most common skin disorders.

- Acne: poor digestion of fats
- Eczema: poor digestion of carbohydrates
- Psoriasis: poor digestion of proteins
- Pimples and blackheads: toxicity overload
- Lipoma: rancid fats buildup
- Cellulite: toxins trapped in fats
- Wrinkled skin: loss of skin elasticity
- Overall poor digestion and lack of water

In addition, almost all skin hives and rashes will respond favorably to enzyme therapy.

THE END OF A CHRONIC CONDITION

A 30-year-old client of mine called Nancy came to me with a moderate but pesky case of psoriasis on her hands, arms, and feet. As a nurse, Nancy needed to wash her hands often during the day, which aggravated the condition and made her daily life very uncomfortable. Before calling me, Nancy had tried several topical medications, skin emollients, steroids, and even a recommended diet change. But nothing noticeably influenced the itchy, scaly skin.

I suggested the same course of enzyme therapy that I followed for my own problem with eczema. She took a multi-enzyme supplement with each meal and a high-dose protease between meals on an empty stomach. After three days of this therapy, Nancy could feel the positive effects of enzymes. Her energy level significantly increased. She noticed her digestive problems with bloating and belching had subsided. One week later, her skin showed marked improvement. The scales began to disappear and the color became more even. The overall appearance of her skin was vibrant and healthy. In 21 days the psoriasis that doctors had told her would be a lifelong condition for her had vanished. Nancy is still on the same enzyme regimen. Her skin problems no longer exist.

YOUTHFUL SKIN

How youthful is your skin? Try the following simple experiment. Pinch the skin on the back with one hand between the thumb and forefinger of the other hand for five seconds. Then let it go and time how long it takes to return to normal. If your skin takes five seconds or less to return to normal, then the biological age of your skin is less than 50. Ten to 15 seconds indicate an age range of 60 to 69. Time exceeding 15 seconds shows the biological age of your skin as 70 or more. It takes longer as we age. This is reflected in the wrinkles we bear from the deterioration of tissue under the surface of the skin.

Many researchers claim that aging skin is often caused by a lack of protein and a weak circulatory system. These deficiencies cause tissue, muscles, nerve fibers, and blood vessels to become rigid. They are responsible for loss of muscle tone and skin elasticity, resulting in sagging and drooping skin as well as muscles. This degenerative process can be slowed and sometimes even reversed with a healthy protein diet and enzyme therapy.

THE PROTEIN CONNECTION

Specialized proteins broken down by protease maintain the integrity of our supporting tissue and furnish normal elasticity for the skin. The interlocking of elastin, a yellow, fibrous protein that is the basic constituent of elastic connective tissue, with collagen in the layers of the skin keeps it smooth and supple. However, as we age, this interlocking system hardens. The aging process is arrested when there is an adequate supply of enzymes to feed the skin, to deliver abundant supplies of oxygen, to keep the cells plump, and to allow the dermis to replenish itself with healthy new skin.

Imagine the cells and tissues of the body looking like a sponge. These cells and tissues need the moisturizing agents delivered by protease in order to function efficiently. When the body's cells lack amino acids delivered by protease, they become thirsty and they atrophy, or waste away because of insufficient nutrition. The characteristics of a sponge disappear. The cells absorb less of the necessary protein and the cellular walls break down, dry, and shrink. By this time, aging has set in.

EFFECTIVE CIRCULATION

The circulatory system as well plays a key role in aging. A sluggish system delays the delivery of needed nutrients to the skin cells. A blood supply that is low in essential nutrients sabotages the needs of the skin to stay healthy. Once again, it is enzymes that will rescue!I emphasize again...Enzymes are the digestive catalysts that make nutrients available to the blood for their journey to every cell in the body.

Lipase enzymes keep off the buildup of plaque and platelets on the walls of the arteries. This allows the blood plasma rich nutrients to provide the proteases, nutrients, and oxygen to get to the cells on schedule. Protease is the life force of the circulatory system and its blood. Protease keeps the blood moving by cleaning up congested red blood cells, which can stick together in clumps. Through microscopic live blood analysis, we can see how after only 10 minutes, one dose of protease immediately loosens sticky cells and frees the blood flow. Because the body is composed of protein, protease feeds and fortifies the cells of the blood itself, making them stronger and better equipped to carry out the task of distributing nutrients.

Because the skin is the largest organ of the body, it is a primary benefactor of an enzyme-rich circulatory system. Skin that is well enriched by oxygen and high quality nutrients always looks radiant, firm, and smooth.

YOUNG SKIN AT 60

At the age of 60, Carl called on me because his gums were bleeding and his front tooth was loose. He had high hopes that enzyme therapy could help his periodontal problems. A high-dose regimen of protease cleared up the swollen and inflamed gums and saved the tooth. He was an avid convert to protease therapy. Not long after starting his enzymes, Carl noticed an unexpected bonus from his daily intake of enzyme supplements—he looked 20 years younger! His skin looked smooth and soft. It lost its wrinkled and hardened appearance. Even its color was youthful. Carl phoned me one day to tell me that people were constantly telling him he looked great. Everyone wanted to know his secret. "I'm tempted to keep it a secret," Carl laughed. "But no one believes me anyway when I tell them I found the fountain of youth in enzymes."

ENZYME THERAPY FOR SKIN

To feed, detoxify and slow the aging process of the skin, you must dedicate yourself to a lifelong program of enzyme therapy. However, a good way to obtain the necessary supply of nutrients is from your foods. I also advise an increase in your intake of foods rich in plant proteins. These include non-GMOs:

brown rice	kasha	seeds
buckwheat	millet	soybeans
bulgur	nuts	wheat germ

It is difficult to get GMO-free soybeans so be very sure they are organic. Raw fruit and vegetable nutrients eaten with the enzyme supplementation are good for the skin. Because protease is the enzyme that is most vital to a healthy skin, you would take it between meals. Ingesting a good plant-based digestive supplement with meals should be added to your program. Giving your body lipase enzymes in the digestive formula will assist in the proper breakdown of fats. You will not have a healthy fatty acid balance without proper lipase taken with meals.

THE SECRETS OF HEALTHY SKIN

The units of activity of enzyme supplements vary from label to label. Those of you with severe skin problems may need very high units that can only be purchased from a health-care professional. In most cases, if you read labels carefully you can find a multi -enzyme supplement with the appropriate units of activity. These unit numbers are the minimum dosage you desire for a successful program.

Take these supplemental plant-based digestive enzymes with food:

- Carbohydrate-splitting enzymes in correct proportions
- Lipase: 2000 LU or higher
- Protease: 65,000 HUT or above

Between meals to fortify and detoxify:

- Systemic blended Protease: 330,000 to 420,000 HUT

The secret to youthful skin is supplemental enzymes. This is not regarded as one of life's great mysteries. It is not complex since all of this information is well-documented, proven, and simple. Your skin needs the continuous nourishment from within that only good nutrition and supplemental enzymes can supply. Remember, the nutrients cannot make it to the skin without their carriers (enzymes).

There are so many success stories I could relate, but then this book would be too heavy for the reader to lift. Psoriasis and other skin disorders clear in short periods of time, once the enzyme therapy has started. One client had a skin disorder that is referred to as "elephantiasis." The enlargement of certain parts of the body, especially the legs and genitals, characterizes this unsightly condition. The surrounding skin hardens and becomes ulcerated. It is caused by obstruction of the lymphatic vessels, often due to infestation by parasites. This poor woman was in a great deal of pain. Two weeks after she began her enzyme therapy, she could see and feel a notable difference. Others commented to her on how much better she seemed. Working with therapeutic supplemental plant-based enzymes is so exciting. I feel truly blessed to be a part of this wonderful healing art. It makes so much sense to me, because I see it work and get to be part of this healing process!

TESTIMONIALS

***"I am attaching before and after pictures** of my daughter. We tried everything... creams, oils, even steroids, but nothing helped. Her class was going to have an end of the year swim party and she was determined that she was not going to go. I tested her using EAV equipment and the protocol called for the protease. She started taking them and literally started healing in two days. By the end of the two weeks, you could not tell that she had psoriasis. She has not had to repeat the protocol. It has been three years and she's totally healed. Thanks for the great products." - SS4H*

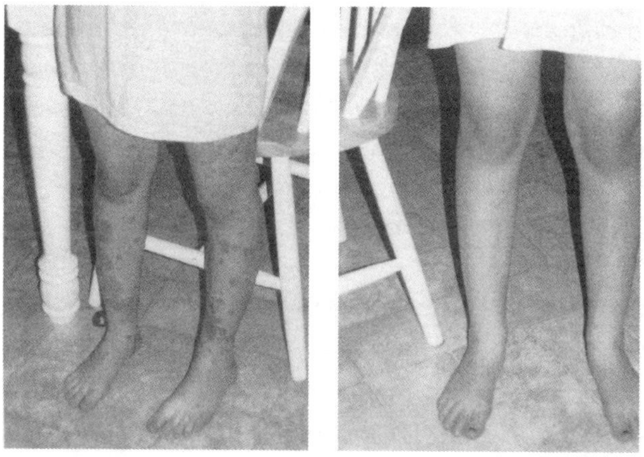

***"I wanted to tell you** about a six-year-old girl that came to me with eczema. She had been to over 10 doctors that said it was the worst case of eczema they had ever seen. It literally covered her entire body. Part of her protocol I gave her was using your protease for sensitives and two homeopathics. It took her about four months to heal but her mother says she has only a little patch on her skin now. They are going to come back to see me soon. Again, thanks for your commitment to excellence." - Rebecca KS*

***"I have shared** the Acne Protocol with some estheticians that asked for it, and I also sent it to my daughter. She is 23 now-how did she get so grown up? She wanted to clear her skin for a magazine photo shoot. Anyway, she texted me today and said her skin is as clear as when she was on birth control pills! She is taking your master endocrine product, Digest, Protease & Probiotic. She has also cleaned up her diet, drinking water and goes to yoga class every other day. I thought you would like to hear that feedback." - Dawn A., CNC*

Re: My wife is no longer planning her funeral!

"My wife had an accident last July in which she fell backwards and broke her wrist. Shortly afterwards she started getting a rash on her body which was treated with anti-histamines. The situation got steadily worse, the rash is now permanent and she is taking the anti-histamine three times a day. We discovered that she was hypothyroid and suffering from adrenal fatigue, suspected that she had developed a food intolerance and "leaky gut" and have been told that this is chronic idiopathic urticaria but now treatment has been offered. Her enzyme protocol now includes your sensitive protocol of a digestive, protease, probiotic and gut soothing enzyme supplements. Her condition has vastly improved. She was taking 10 mg anti-histamine three times a day and now reduced to 5 mg once only, with minimal rashes appearing in the morning. And they do not last long before disappearing. Her general outlook has also improved. She is no longer planning her funeral!!! The sparkle is back and she looks and feels good. And she has lost 20 pounds, down to a size 12. Coincidently, this morning was the first day that absolutely no rash appeared." - Robbie P., MD - United Kingdom

***"I couldn't wait for Monday** to call and tell you that my son's acne is like 75 percent better. He had it all over his face. I am so happy and he is too—as excited as an 18-year-old boy can be. I just emailed one of my new clients and told her I can hardly wait to start the protocol. She also has a lot of acne and has been on medication with no real improvements. I just want to thank your clinic and the staff for being so patient with all my questions and me. I love being able to share the knowledge and help people to change their lifestyles to live a healthier life, through prevention." - Jan D.*

***"This is where I believe protease** has been the miracle worker for me. A year ago last October, I was diagnosed with very early stage lichen Sclerosis. I've totally changed what I put in and on my body, and have spent a year detoxifying. Your protease has been a key player in my* *recovery. I saw my doctor just a few weeks ago, and she has confirmed that my lichen Sclerosis is 100 percent gone. There is no evidence that I ever had it. In addition, a body composition analysis shows all of my numbers are right on target, right where they are supposed to be. My blood work also turned out excellent. I am grateful beyond words. Thank you again and again!" - Ginny C.*

"Ten years ago *I had gone through some stress when I lost my Aunt to leukemia. I developed a rash around my thighs inside and out, on my stomach and some on my arms. It was so itchy that I was unable to sleep at night. I scratched day and night. I had gone to see my GP, my allergist, and a Dermatologist. They prescribed steroid pills, expensive cortisone creams, and body washes to no avail. I was so tired of it. I had just read The Healing Power of Enzymes and located the phone number to contact them. Lisa Helffrich answered my call. She asked me what the problem was and I told her. She said, "Well let's see... how far away are you and how soon could you be here"? She was kind enough to see me that day! She took a blood sample and began to help me understand what I needed to start taking. She told me it would probably take 3-4 weeks before I would feel relief. I started taking them that day and within 5-6 days I was already clearing up. I felt immediate relief and my skin cleared as though I never had a problem with my skin. I felt so good that I had forgotten how miserable I had felt. Now I am a true believer of healing with enzymes. I still take some of the enzymes and can tell the difference when I stop taking them. When I get off of enzymes I begin to feel sluggish and tired. I feel much better when I am on enzymes from Dr. DicQie." - Mona H.*

Chapter 15

To A Longer, Healthier & Youthful Life

LONGEVITY POTENTIAL

Aging can be delayed. Tests conducted by Dr. Howell and his colleagues clearly demonstrate that aging and debilitated metabolic enzyme activities are synonymous. Let's make an observation between a healthy human cell and the chemicals that make it. The earth that we live on has its own 94 chemicals, and we have 27 of those chemicals in every one of our cells. Our cell has its 27 chemicals with its 20,000 enzymes and between them they create over 100,000 different chemical actions every second of our lives. To do this they require 45 nutrients from the carbohydrates, fats, and proteins we consume.

If our digestive tract, and the immune system which houses in it, are healthy, then we can properly feed our cells. Other very exciting research continues to shed new light on how our bodies rid themselves of damaged and aging cells. This offers renewed hope that someday we will be able to manipulate these processes in order to further delay aging. That's right, there is growing evidence, including a new study from the British Journal of Sports Medicine, that shows maintaining fitness through middle age could delay biological aging by 12 years.

Think about it. What is far more important to doctors is someone's physiological age. After all, we probably all know 50-year olds who have the health of a 40-year old and unfortunately, vice-versa. This particular study shows exercise, such as jogging and/or walking improves the body's oxygen consumption and its ability to generate energy. That in turns leads to the slowing and possible reversal of the inevitable decline of the body's function. We can, for all intents and purposes, become biologically younger.

I want to submit my biggest positive impression on the aging process, and that is the supplementation of digestive enzymes healthy bacteria (probiotics) to maintain a healthy gut environment. Last but not least are supplemental systemic protease enzymes for balanced inflammation and proper circulation of our blood. Free radicals kill the cells and cause aging. Proteolytic and Lipolytic enzymes rid the body of free radicals. Protease is the major one that creates glutathione in the cells and fights against aging.

FREE RADICALS AND AGING

What are free radicals? Why are they damaging to the human body? In addition, how do enzymes along with other antioxidants help protect the body against free radical damage? With age comes increasing and sometimes cumulative exposure to both natural and synthetic environmental toxins, from heavy metals and pesticides to tobacco smoke and radiation—even life-giving oxygen can be harmful. Much of the damage from these exposures results from the generation of "free radicals." These extremely reactive molecules or fragments of molecules have unpaired, or "free," electrons that in the normal course of metabolism are channeled into energy production. In some cells, they may be used to kill viruses and bacteria. However, because of their extremely high energy and inexorable search for another electron, they can also damage normal tissues if too many are produced or are not adequately controlled. The prematurely aged, wrinkled skin of smokers is caused by the free radical-induced damage that smoking creates. In fact, smoking is probably the greatest source of voluntary exposure to free radicals.

In our bloodstream, they will steal an electron from any atom, without discrimination. This creates another free radical, and another and another... soon, a good deal of damage is done and the body's health really begins to falter. When we observe this using live blood under the microscope, we find the platelets clumped together, forming thrombocytes (blood clotting). When the body or artery is under attack, thrombocytes rush to the trouble spot and form clumps. This creates a blood flow problem. In addition, the body naturally makes a fiber-like protein found in the plasma as well. Then, the appropriate minerals are dispatched to the aggravated site. If calcium is sent, it reacts to the area under siege and forms its own type of plaque. This can result in various signs of aging, such as loss of memory, hearing, vision, and stamina. Oxidative stress also inactivates critical enzymes and other proteins.

Natural protection: The body produces essential antioxidant defenses internally. Enzymes that control free radicals include superoxide dismutase, glutathione peroxidase, and catalase, as well as other molecules such as cholesterol, steroid hormones and sulfur-containing amino acids that neutralize free radicals. It is also possible to choose many nutrients in both foods and supplements that help fight free radicals. Most free radical protection involves eating a better diet, exercising, maintaining a clean environment both internally and externally, and reducing stress, in addition to taking enzyme supplements.

BIOLOGICALLY YOUNGER

I've also learned how important upper-body training is, for both men and women. Simply adding some upper body strength leads to increased muscle mass, improved bone density and increased lung capacity—all-important things to extend life. Do you have some other ideas? Forget for one second about simply looking younger—how do you think we can become biologically younger today?

There are ways to measure biological aging and that is by measuring the ratio of your muscle to your fat with a Body Comp Analysis (BCA). If you have healthy fluids and enough muscle for health compared to a lower fat, you would show a rating that puts you in a younger category. The general overview of this information plus your actual height and weight will give a biological age, which has nothing to do with your chronological age. The thrill of being an age of 70 but given a biological age of 50 certainly helps you continue your healthy process.

IS THERE A DRUG TO LIVE LONGER? YES, IF YOU ARE A FAT MOUSE!

Normally, the body clears out old cells, but the process becomes less efficient with age. So researchers at the Mayo Clinic used a drug to target only senescent cells (cells that loose power of division and growth) and force them to self-destruct in a group of mice that were genetically engineered to age rapidly. In mice that were treated throughout their lifetimes, researchers said they saw a remarkable delay in the development of cataracts, muscle wasting, and the type of fat loss that causes skin wrinkling in humans. Another group of mice was treated in older age after cataracts had already set in. The drug didn't reverse the age-related changes that had already occurred, but it prevented further decline. In modern medicine, aging is sometimes considered a disease just like any other. Since people unsurprisingly want to live longer, healthier lives, the question becomes whether it's possible to delay aging. The answer is: **Kill all the sickly old cells!**

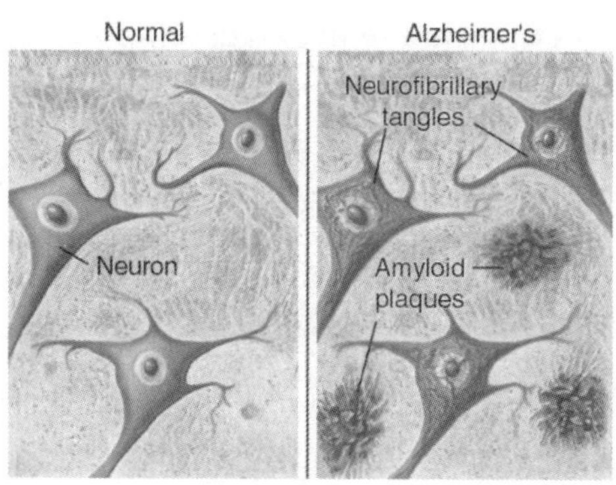

In the meantime, we already have some fascinating information about the role enzymes play. When taken between meals to work in the blood system, protease enzymes remove excessive proteins from our system and these can be the sickly old cells.

We know that the major cause of aging is cellular deterioration due to excess toxins in the body. This in turn reflects a weakened immune system from the destruction of free radicals causing a general contamination of the blood. I find it very interesting that nearly every problem or adverse condition hinges on virtually the same deficiencies. In the previous chapter you learned how current studies on plant-based enzyme supplementation cause the skin to look more youthful.

I ask my elderly clients (I find this funny since I am 70 years old) to adopt an anti-aging stance, and then attack with gusto! It is simply not enough to eat well and exercise.

- Everyone has to add nutrients to his or her diet, preferably in herbal, freeze dried foods to provide nutrients from foods
- Everyone has to get enough sleep—around eight hours
- Everyone has to take time each day to meditate, pray, or spend time in a relaxed state remembering to take deep breaths
- Everyone has to eat those foods that are appropriate for his or her genetic biochemical type
- Everyone has to take supplemental plant-based enzymes with meals to digest food and between meals to repair the system. We stop making metabolic digestive enzymes as we age. Science tells us that proteases are first released to properly break down proteins.
- Those who faithfully remain on their plans tell me they have never felt better or more energized since they were kids. That is because, first and foremost, a good program of enzyme supplements helps your body get the most out of the foods you eat.
- By fortifying and revitalizing your organs and tissues, you achieve balanced health and anti-aging support.
- Supplemental plant-based digestive enzymes and supplemental plant based systemic protease enzymes assist the body to heal itself.

WHY ENZYMES KEEP THE BODY FEELING YOUNGER

After reviewing results from a variety of tests on aging, Dr. Edward Howell, who began his study of enzymes in 1930, concluded: "Humans eating an enzyme-less diet use up a tremendous amount of their enzyme potential in lavish secretions of the pancreas and other digestive organs. The result is a shortened life span (65 years or less as compared with 100 or more), illness, and lowered resistance to stresses of all types, psychological and environmental. By eating foods and supplementing cooked foods with enzyme capsules, we can stop abnormal and pathological aging processes." My favorite quotation from the work of Dr. Howell is: "If you take in enzyme reinforcements during the younger years, your enzymes at 80 years will be more like those at 40 years." Aging has a great deal to do with decreased enzyme reserves. Enzyme therapy slows down the aging process by building up the enzyme reserves and quenching free radicals.

Anytime we suffer from an acute or chronic illness, it is almost certain enzyme depletion exists.

Those with digestive disturbances, endocrine gland imbalances, blood sugar imbalances, diabetes, obesity, high cholesterol, high triglycerides, and stress-related problems will need supplemental enzymes. Supplemental protein enzymes aid in helping your body with detoxifying. They free up more metabolic enzyme energy to enhance detoxification. If you have a very busy life, fly or travel a great deal, and cannot eat those foods common to the area where you live, your enzyme reserves are even more depleted.

DNA DETERIORATION & AGING

Did you know that as we age our DNA deteriorates very quickly? In some individuals this means they can lose approximately 1,000 miles a day of their DNA. Don't panic. Your DNA, if unwound, would stretch out to reach the sun (over 93 million miles from earth and back) approximately 200 times. I have a greater respect for God's greatest creation.

This deterioration reduces enzyme production, which can produce severe changes in our chemistry, which lead to several diseases. This deterioration can be slowed by proper nutrition, enzyme supplementation, and absorption of the 45 required nutrients at the cell, exercise, and good stress reduction in our lifestyles.

HOW LACK OF ENZYMES SPEEDS THE AGING PROCESS

Medicine has discovered little about how to retard the inexorable process of aging. Biologists do not even agree on its definition. We do know that cells tend to die off faster than they can be replaced. After the age of 25, the body's water content and energy reserves noticeably begin to decline. Body efficiency decreases roughly by one percent per year. Tissues waste away, enzymes disappear, mutations damage the genes and organs wear out, one after another. Typically, in the body of an 80-year-old man, 50 million cells are dying each second, while perhaps only 30 million new ones replace them. His muscles have lost 30 percent of their former weight, his brain has shriveled by 10 percent, and nerve trunks have shed 25 percent of their fibers. Each breath takes in 50 percent less oxygen, each heartbeat pumps 35 percent less blood, the blood absorbs oxygen 60 percent more slowly, and the kidneys, loyal team members that they are, have sacrificed their efficiency by half to help other organs worse off than themselves.

That our bodies continue to function in spite of all this, speaks wonders for this biological miracle of 100 organs, 200 bones, 600 muscles and over one trillion cells! To carry on a detailed discussion of the way all these parts work would bewilder the reader and me. It is sufficient to know that none of these parts or processes can possibly work without enzymes. Enzymes are the energy and substances that make life possible. They are a necessary component of every chemical action that takes place in the human body. The truth is we should eat for our cells and they will keep us healthy if they are healthy.

Invariably any discussion about enzymes results in the question: Do we lose our ability to produce enzymes because we age, or do we age because our ability to sustain production of enzymes decreases? My thought is "who cares?"...let's just replace them with supplemental plant-based enzymes. If we were to take too many of which I certainly doubt, then they just help make more metabolic enzymes because they are proteins. Proteins (amino acids) help the body produce metabolic enzymes.

TESTIMONIAL

"I am not sure how these enzyme supplements work, but I know what they do for me. I have been on them faithfully for 18 years, and I am not going to stop taking them. I am 72 years old and am not on any medication. I have regular checkups and all lab tests are normal. My energy is nonstop and I still work fulltime. My life is good, and I credit it to these supplements DicQie has me on. In fact, when many of my friends comment on my health I tell them about the enzymes, however if they complain about their own health I send them to DicQie."

Chapter 16

Enzymes and Your Pet's Health

THE IMPORTANCE OF ENZYMES IN YOUR PET'S DIET

Our pets don't deserve to eat one meal without enzymes. The foods that we feed our pets are processed, canned, cooked, and nutritionally damaged in some way. Remember, processing food or heating food above 118 degrees will destroy the nutritional activity. This is the reason why our pets have all the same digestive disorders and diseased conditions that people have.

Whenever pet owners or my Veterinarian friends ask me how they can support their pet's overall health, we tell them to look at the very first step—digestion. Your pet depends on his or her digestive tract to supply the necessary enzymes required to digest food and to perform countless metabolic functions throughout his or her body. But if the necessary enzymes aren't there, your pet may suffer from occasional abdominal discomfort, gas, and vomiting. But that's not all; insufficient digestive enzymes can affect their overall health too. You may not realize it, but important functions like detoxification, joint movement, skin and oral health, and immune function all depend on enzymes for both our bodies and their bodies.

Just about any food you feed your pet today—whether it's processed dry, canned, high quality frozen, or even homemade raw food—may not be adequately digested because his or her body may not be able to supply all the enzymes for digestion. Pets are carnivores and their bodies may not recognize some foods. If that is the case, then the nutrients do not get to the cells that the pet potentially needs. All the nutrients in commercial pet foods are synthetic, which means only a part can be absorbed. Therefore, I believe that just about all cats and dogs can benefit from a supplemental digestive enzyme to support their optimal digestion and health. In fact, pets normally do not have a choice in the foods they are fed.

Dogs digest their foods just as humans do. Cats have more of a digestive problem due to the breed's improper fat digestion, which leads to their kidney problems. Dogs and cats require digestive enzymes since their food is broken down in the same digestive pattern. We humans can tell someone when we hurt or have poor digestion, but our pets can't. It shows up as constipation, diarrhea, itchy skin, and shedding of their fur until it turns into a disease. Just like humans, they inherit an enzyme potential that is dependent on their own unique DNA. Add the genetic problems in breeding of the animals, and you compound their predicament.

Enzyme deficiency may be the primary reason for many of the problems existing in veterinary concerns today. In the early days of my business and clinical research, we had several doctors on our board and most are still with the company today. One of my special board members is Dr. Todd Robeck, and he is affiliated with Sea World because of his specialty as a veterinarian and a fertility specialist. It was fun because when we wanted to see Todd we could visit Sea World and he would let us behind the scenes. This was the first time I had arranged to visit Sea World to meet him along with another doctor and his two friends. Todd introduced me to the killer whales and a sweet dolphin named Lucky. Lucky had eczema on one side of his body and was very shy. Of course, having suffered with it myself, my heart went out to him.

Todd called me one day saying they were having problems with one of their killer whales and his blood work was showing serious kidney problems. He asked how much protease he would need to give the whale. I asked how many tons he weighs. I had no idea on how to determine dosage, so we settled on protease in a fish and went from there. I do not know if you have ever seen the size of capsules they use, but you could stand in one! I arranged to get him our protease blend in kilos, and we struggled with the amount but did something right because the killer whale lived.

They invited me up to show them how the protease can work effectively in the blood by using my microscope, but I was in London teaching so my sister-in-law Jeannie went in my place with our microscope in tow. It is very rare for them to grant nutritionals or much of anything used on these extremely valuable creatures. We were given permission by Sea World in San Antonio to speak about the use of enzymes, but I did not know how to relate the story about eczema and killer whales or dolphins. What followed was an invitation to speak to doctors in Dubai about enzymes for animals, and I asked Todd to go in my place. I knew they raised horses, which were expensive commodities. He did a beautiful job, and they showed him their surgical rooms for the horses. Todd has gone on to become famous in Sea World circles around the world because he was able to use his fertility magic for births of killer whales in captivity.

Dr. Robert Turesky, a research scientist for the Division of Environmental Health Sciences at the New York State Department of Health, had done a study on hair analysis to detect the presence of specific carcinogens in cooked meat. As a test, Dr. Turesky analyzed the fur of his own dogs and to his surprise, discovered the presence of one of the carcinogens he was researching. Since his dogs don't eat grilled steaks or burgers, it seemed clear they were being exposed through their own processed pet food diet.

Veterinarian Karen Becker discovered that, including Dr. Turesky's published study, there appears to be only two studies in existence that address the potential for carcinogenic substances in processed pet food. When we consider the fact that most dogs and cats eat commercial processed diets during their entire lives, and when we also take into account the escalating incidence of cancer in pets – especially dogs – it seems this topic deserves more attention. Based on Dr. Turesky's findings on carcinogen levels in cooked poultry-based protein sources, and to what we know about the extreme processing dry pet food undergoes, it seems the worst thing you can feed your beloved dog or cat is a poultry-based dry food. As always, fresh raw, freeze-dried or air-dried meat-based diets, well balanced, are Dr. Becker's recommendation for healthy dogs and cats.

Nature intended for the enzymes in food to assist the natural digestive enzymes secreted by the animal. If food is not digested as nature planned, it cannot supply an animal with the nutrition needed to build and repair vital organs and tissue, produce energy, and maintain a strong immune defense system. Enzyme synergy and cell metabolism are important for complete utilization of the potential nutritive value of foods. In the absence of active enzymes in food, the foodstuffs may lead to diseases for our beloved animals.

Research has shown that animals in the wild have much less chronic degenerative disease than domesticated animals.

This can be directly attributable to their food sources. When animals are fed with cooked, canned, dried, or any of the processed food stuffs, the responsibility for digestion falls entirely on the animal's digestive system. This compromises their immune system. When a supplemental plant-based, multi-enzyme formulation is added to the animal's diet, the same enzymatic activity is available for digestion that is needed to handle the processed foods. This relieves some of the burden placed on the digestive and immune systems.

An enzyme/nutrient-deficient diet may lead to musculoskeletal inflammation, a major cause of discomfort and debility in millions of older canines. Osteoarthritis, loss of mobility and movement, pain, and swelling can be relieved with enzyme supplementation. Relief from edema, a major source of irritation for an animal, has also been experienced.

Protease enzymes break down protein foods. When taken between meals, protease enzymes hydrolyze large protein molecules into smaller polypeptides and amino acids. When larger protein molecules (bacteria, cellular debris, parasites, and fungal forms) are hydrolyzed and become soluble, they are more readily passed in the urine. Protease clears inflammation from the system. Lipase enzymes aid in proper fat and lipid digestion. When taken between meals, it also provides essential fatty acids to maintain skin, coat, and other tissues. Carbohydrate-splitting enzymes assist in the breaking down of carbohydrates. If carbohydrates are not properly digested, they cannot be used for energy. When taken in between meals, they aid in the control of inflammation caused as a result of poor digestion.

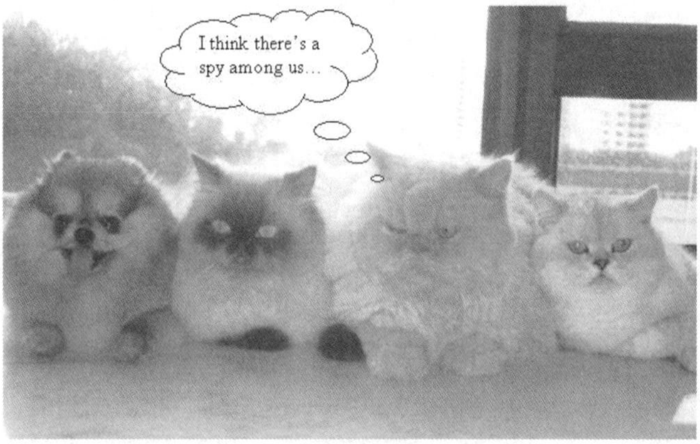

CASE HISTORY

Dr. Jim Smith, a veterinarian specializing in animal allergy and dermatological problems, has been performing clinical research with supplemental plant-based enzymes. He was thrilled with the results and says the time expected for healing response is not just cut in half, but in many cases in 72 hours. This of course depends on the condition of the animal. But in all the years of his practice, he has not seen anything in medicine or any other supplement work like the enzyme protease for mange, foot biting, mites, parasites, ear infections, and various other conditions that he sees on an ongoing basis in his clinics. Dr. Smith has been working with other veterinarians by teaching veterinarian enzyme therapy usage.

Vets using the enzymes have seen amazing results with large animals such as horses and even the very large elephants. The challenge for me has been to come up with some of the dosages. This has been real education for me. Most of the doctors tell me that 50 percent and higher of the ailments that bring animals to their clinics are directly related to diet and nutritional imbalances. These particular animals have a different digestive system, so the time for enzymes used for digestion is planned for the animal. This is not an area of my expertise, but all I can do is use common sense in trying to direct the traffic in digestion and enzyme therapy.

What enzymes have done for the health of the animal kingdom is exactly the same as for the human race. I know that by now you surely have some usable information about enzymes for the health of your family and your pets. But please remember the best way is the preventative way. However, if you have a condition, it is important for you to educate yourself and look at all possible choices.

According to PetfoodIndustry.com, a major industry player is losing market share because consumers are "increasingly choosing pet foods that more closely resemble their own foods." It seems more and more pet owners are actively seeking out smaller pet food companies that sell products with higher quality ingredients. The pet food industry as a whole is undergoing a shift in response to consumer demand for the same types of ingredients and foods for their pets that they want for themselves. Pet owners are looking for products and ingredients that are (or are perceived to be) natural, fresh and locally sourced (or at least not sourced from, for example, China). According to the Wall Street Journal, "The image of lab-engineered nutrition like Hill's has become a liability in an age where the new mark of quality is organic or natural, and the brand has lost market share."

When I cannot fix proper foods for my two Vizsla dogs, I pay money in proportion to what I get. Right now I am purchasing Evangers Gold Label. I give my dogs supplemental plant-based digestive enzymes, proper probiotics, and added protease. Our dogs live long and our oldest Vizsla named Rascal was 18 human years when he passed. I wonder how long he would have lived with quality of life had I married his owner earlier in this precious dog's life.

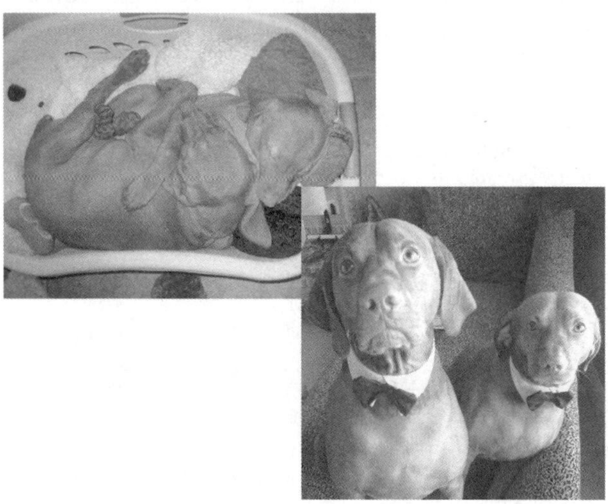

Plant-based digestive enzymes come in capsules or powder so you can decide which fits your pet's palate. Cats seem to prefer the powder taken out of the capsule; some dogs just eat the capsules mixed in their food. My sister-in-law just tosses the enzymes to her dogs and they eat them as if they were given a treat.

One of our dogs named Max will take enzymes anyway he can get them, yet his brother, Buddy, likes the powder and will not eat the capsules. They are from the same litter but their preferences are similar, yet different. If there is a dog biochemical type Buddy has problems with fats (Type Two) and Max has problems with carbohydrates (Type One). I try to give them protein foods as an ongoing regimen but cannot always control our family and friends treating them.

TESTIMONIAL

Re: tremendous success in my veterinary practice

"Just wanted to take a moment to let you know how wonderful your products are. I have had tremendous success in particular with two of your products in my veterinary practice: your gastrointestinal formula and Probiotic. The products are very gentle and well tolerated even by small 3 lb. pets. I use the Gastro and Probiotic (dosages vary depending upon size of pet) for cats and dogs with irritable bowel syndrome and any type of gastrointestinal distress. Just recently, I adopted a beautiful white husky named Blue who had waited for two years to get a home because he has severe irritable bowel syndrome and pancreatitis. I have had to proceed very slowly with him because any change causes a reaction—even if it is a change for the better. Blue was belching and regurgitating most of the night even though he was on special food for a sensitive stomach. I introduced the Probiotic and saw immediate results—he slept through the night comfortably and his loose stool firmed up. This is not a one-time incident. I hear from many cat and dog owners that these two products have helped their pets' loose stool and tummy rumbling almost instantaneously. I have tried other manufacturers and have not found the same results. Thank you!!!!" - Susan D., CCN

Chapter 17

The Athlete Performance & Recovery

ENZYMES STRENGTHEN AND REPAIR YOUR MUSCLES

Enzymes may be the most important, but also the most neglected, essential element of vibrant health. In fact, enzymes may be what make the difference between our fit, young, Olympic athletes and those youth who choose a path of sluggishness. Body builders have a special appreciation of enzymes. If muscle tissue enzymes were not at work, there would be no growth of new muscles. No neurological responses would occur to make the muscle work at all. Enzymes are the catalyst that transforms food into the necessary energy to make muscles move and grow. Because oxygen is one of the sources of enzyme production, proper breathing and exercise are very important for enzyme metabolism.

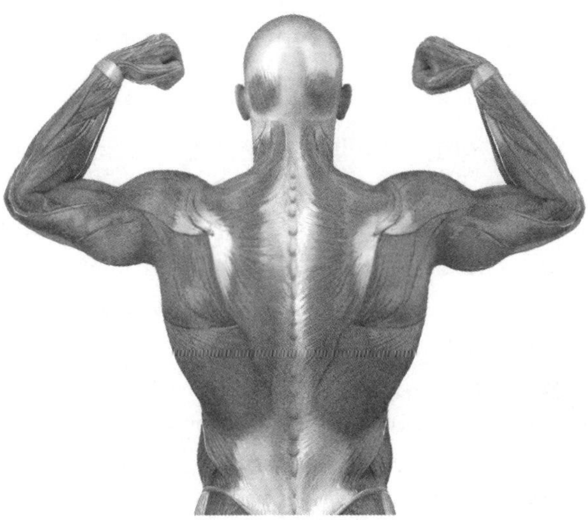

Natural exercise, like walking, helps generate metabolic enzymes. If you are not doing regular, healthy exercise, you will probably have an enzyme deficiency. Creation of enzymes is diminished with disuse of the muscular system. I am not referring to strenuous exercise or weight lifting. I favor exercise that is natural to the human body, like walking, swimming, or bicycling. Scientists are now showing a greater interest in nutrition than ever before. Still, very few have discovered the most important and invigorating factor in a truly potent diet—Enzymes. We are all our own living, breathing pharmacies. Each of us carries a built in fountain of youth. To turn it on and keep it perpetually running, do what it takes to step up production of metabolic enzymes.

The feeding of muscle cells requires 45 nutrients. These must be delivered to those cells by enzymes. If you desire to build muscles or take part in an active fitness program beyond natural exercise, these 45 essential nutrients must be provided along with protease enzymes. If these nutritional components that increase stamina are not created, disastrous results may ensue. Many people have attempted to build their bodies and have experienced nothing but greater fatigue. This is an indication that you are lacking enzymes in your system. Enzymes occur naturally in every living cell. Without them, there would be no life. We must find a way to continually refurbish our bodies.

We have ample proof that we lose enzymes in our perspiration. I have analyzed the blood of many athletes. Those who run or constantly "overdo" tend to have some of the worst blood I have ever seen. Exercise helps in the removal of waste from our system. That is, a moderate, healthy amount of exercise that works in our favor. There is such a thing as over-exercising in which the body begins to break itself down. Two forms of exercise that help to remove toxins are brisk walking several times per week or perhaps a cardiovascular workout at a local club three times per week. These generate metabolic enzymes. Be cautious and always strive for balance in all facets of your life.

Enzymes transfer the energy resulting from good, complete digestion to the muscles, nerves, bones, and glands. This helps in the reduction of swelling and inflammation. These "wonder drugs of nature" build muscle and enhance muscle movement and coordination. They maintain sharp memory, mental well-being, and physiological stability. They afford us protection from the hazards of environmental pollution and other toxins to which we are constantly exposed. Without enzymes, we could not exhale carbon dioxide when we breathe. Any interruption or corruption of these vital functions would be disastrous. Imagine how our health would suffer if we could not produce energy or build and repair tissue and muscle. We would be rendered helpless and our bodies would decay. Many diseases attack us when we lose these enzymes. It is a known fact that if we exercise or exert our bodies beyond the fuel we have available to us, catabolism sets in. This breaks down muscle and tissue, leaving us in a far worse position than we were before we began our exercise program.

INCREASE MUSCLE STRENGTH

If your goal is to increase muscle strength, beware of some high protein drinks and high carbohydrate energy bars. Because these products contain large quantities of sugars along with quickly absorbed proteins, the circulatory system becomes sticky due to the excess protein in the bloodstream. This stickiness keeps the blood cells from delivering oxygen to the tissues. To remedy this, supplemental enzymes will help in the digestion of these drinks and bars. High dosages of protease between meals will break down the excessive protein content in the blood and even assist to build muscle faster. Usually the enzymes added to the product are just enough to possibly deliver the product, which may be doubtful, but not enough to clean up the system from the easily absorbed proteins and carbohydrates (glucose).

TESTIMONIAL

Tim Brown is a Heisman Trophy winner and one of the NFL's most prolific wide receivers, a nine-time Pro Bowl selection in 16 seasons with the Los Angeles Raiders where he holds franchise records for touchdowns, receiving yards, and punt return yards. An analyst for Fox Sports Network, Comcast's Pro Football Now, and News America since his retirement, Tim is also heavily involved in the "9-1-1 for Kids" emergency preparedness program, is an ambassador to the President's Physical Fitness Council on Behalf of Reebok, and is starting a NASCAR racing team as part of their "Drive for Diversity" program.

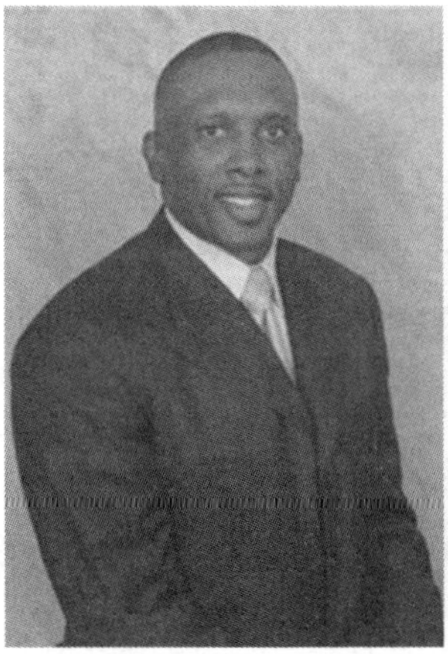

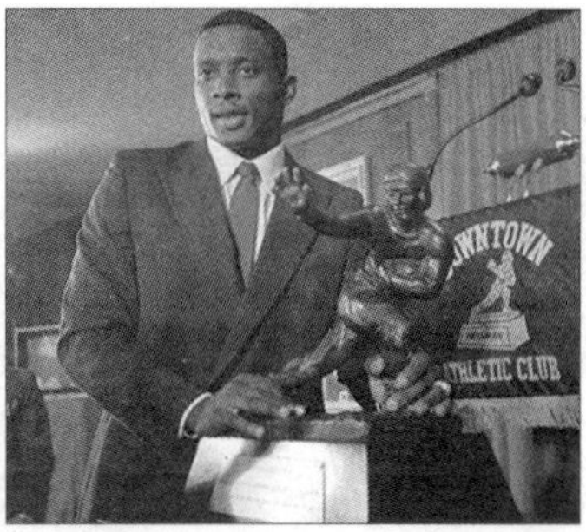

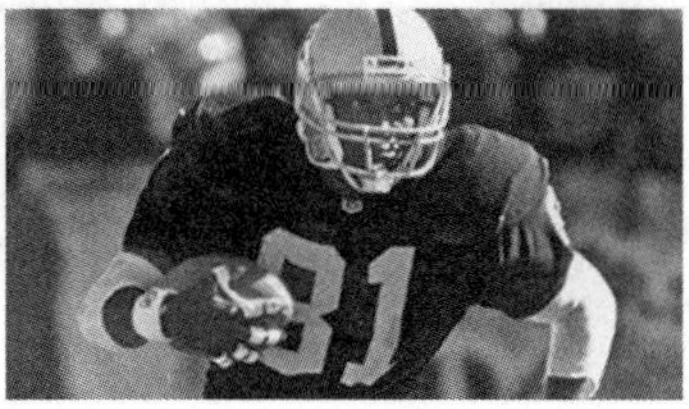

In my 17 years in the NFL, I was one of those guys who did whatever the doctor said to do. I never took any vitamins; I never took anything that was healthy. I tore my knee up in 1989, my second year in the league,

so I literally lived on Indocin for the next 15 years. I knew that Indocin would hurt my liver or my kidneys, but I didn't go a day without taking Indocin until I met Dr. Fuller.

I hurt my thumb in 2004, my last year in the NFL, when I was playing with the Tampa Bay Buccaneers. It was the same thumb I had hurt three years prior, and I had played 10 weeks of the season with two fingers taped together because the thumb was inflamed. So I took five protease right after practice, then I took five later on that night. Long story short, the problem that had stuck with me for three months, three years prior was literally gone in 48 hours. When I was getting ready to go out to practice two days after I started taking enzymes, the doctor was about to tape my thumb up, and he thought I had gotten a shot in my thumb, because all of a sudden I had no more pain in my thumb. And for me, that was amazing. That was one of the first times I realized that, okay, I've got something special here.

Another problem I had at the time was from my surgeries. And one of the things I noticed immediately when I'd taken Protease is that I didn't have that stiffness in my body when I sat down and got up. My joints weren't aching and nothing was tight. I didn't have any issues anymore when I got up in the morning either. And to me, that was mind-blowing. I was about 37-years-old and my body is feeling better than when I was 17,18-years-old. And I believe I owe that all to the enzymes. My ability to move around, to feel great, to play with my kids, to do all those things—things I didn't know five years ago if I'd be able to do. I feel a lot more confident now that I'll be okay.

I don't take anything else. My daily regimen is Protease in the morning when I get up, then Protease IFC, ExcellZyme and Super CellZyme. And I'll repeat that process probably about two to three o'clock in the afternoon. Of course I carry Digest and EFA's in my pocket—I don't go anywhere without those. Then at night I'll do the same thing, and I may add a couple of Gastro when I go to bed. And that has been my life. For the last four years I take nothing—I take no Advil, I take no Claritin D, no inflammation pills, nothing. I live with enzymes. And I say I live 'with' enzymes, not 'on' enzymes. I'm living with them and they have been, and I think will continue to be, great for me as I move on.

Now I'm the enzyme man—that's what my wife calls me, "the enzyme man." I was just amazed that the whole world didn't know about it. I was shocked that the whole world did not know about Dr. DicQie and the enzyme program that they have. So immediately I wanted to get everybody involved, to get other players involved in it, and to get my family involved. As much as I possibly can, I'm talking to everybody I run into who I think can benefit from this, and we're trying to get in front of as many people as we can.

And that's the great thing about this program. It's not that they're telling you to stop taking what the doctor says. All Dr. DicQie says is to add to whatever you are currently taking. And now in my house, if you have an issue and you're not taking enzymes, I don't want to hear about it. That's just bottom line. I don't care what the doctor said. And I tell you, everyone in my family knows, if you're not taking the enzymes, don't come to the table with any problem you have. If anything comes up, I don't want to hear about it if you're not taking the enzymes.

Everybody at my church knows. My pastor is 72-years-old and both he and his wife are health nuts who eat right and do all the healthy things, and they know about the enzymes and take the enzymes. And if he asks me to come speak at the church, he'll say, "Isn't it amazing? This guy plays 17 years in the NFL, he can still walk straight, he can still walk without limping."

Because in the world that I come from, I'm seeing athletes really just deteriorate as they go on in their life because of what we did for so long. I mean, sure I played 17 years in the NFL, but I played 27 years of football if you go back to junior high, high school, and college. And that can't be good for your body. But I'm glad to know now that after all the harm that I did to my body, hopefully now I'm doing some good for my body. And I really don't think that would be possible without enzymes.

Five years ago if you had this conversation with me about my future and where I thought I would be, I probably wouldn't have been too optimistic. Because all I have is the history that has gone on before me, and the guys whom I know are struggling. I lived in a world where I see guys taking this, taking that, and it's only causing more and more problems for them. They take these anti-inflammatory products, they take products for depression, they take all this stuff, and it's only causing them more and more problems.

I was in a meeting just two or three weeks ago with the Commissioner of the NFL, the Executive Director of the Player's Union, and some older players were in the room. They were talking about all these great things they're going to do for the players as they come out of the league. They're saying, "Well we've got this drug for them, we've got that drug for them, we've got this and we've got that." And I raised my hand and said, "It's only going to cause more problems. You have a drug for the symptom, and when the symptom hits you'll say, 'oh we have a drug for that too. When that symptom hits, we've got a drug for that too.' But before we get to that point, can't we give these guys something that's helpful to them? Do we have any homeopathic methods? You know, is anybody talking about anything that's all natural?" And I get calls now almost on a weekly basis saying, "My back is hurting. I'm tired of taking all this stuff, it's not helping. I hear you've got something going on that's working."

So I'm pushing it on all levels. And part of our business plan is that we want to introduce products to kids—because my four year old twins take them. They get up in the morning, they go down to have breakfast, and they say, "Where are the enzymes?" My son calls them 'zymes. "Where the 'zymes at, daddy? Where the 'zymes at?" They don't walk out of the house without taking their enzymes. And my son has asthma so we take everything. They take PureZyme, they take GastroZyme and they take DigestZyme. Bottom line is they're taking them and they're helpful to them.

Again, my father's 72-years-old, and you know how these old guys from Louisiana who don't listen to anybody about anything are. But now we have him on Digest, EFA's and Protease—he's taking everything. It took me a while to get him on them but now when I go over there, he's shaking his bottle. That means it's time to load up and give him some more. He calls Digest his "tummy pills." He'll say, "Can you bring me those tummy pills? They make my tummy feel good, man."

I could go on because I have tons and tons of stories. About a month and a half ago I burned myself really bad, and in about two weeks it started to fade and fade. And it's literally gone now—you probably can't really see it because it's almost gone. And I told my wife, "Call Dr. DicQie. I don't know what happened. I can't explain why I'm healing like that."

Last Christmas at my place in Dallas, I was climbing up on a ladder because our tree is 15 feet tall. So I'm climbing up to put this tree together, and I smashed my hand and I cut deep into it. And now you can't even tell where that mark is. I have another cut near it back from my basketball days. I got caught up on the rim and cut my finger 10,

12 years ago and this was still there but the one I did last Christmas is absolutely gone. Dr. DicQie maybe can explain it, I can't. But I know it happened and I know it's now gone. And since I'm not taking anything but these enzymes it has to be because of them. Again, that's my testimony.

Thank you. Tim Brown, 10/13/07

Tim is a dear friend of mine and he has honored me by calling me his "white mama." He said I did not give birth to him but I did give him a new life. He still is taking enzymes and talking them up wherever he is. I was at the Heisman Trophy gala last December and he introduced me to several of his friends and just had to talk about enzymes.

OTHER TESTIMONIALS

"I have been a competitive athlete my entire life, and have been a professional strength athlete since 2003. As a result, doctor visits and various treatments have always been part of what I do. I was diagnosed with Spondylolisthesis several years ago and throughout the years have had incurred muscle, tendon and ligament damage on various occasions. Most recently a torn hip flexor hampered me for two competitive seasons, and only recently was I able to once again compete at 100%. The therapy that I receive is unique in that various methods are used to work toward healing. We have had great success with regular adjustments, Active Release, Soft Tissue Mobilization, and most recently customized enzyme therapy with the help of Transformation Enzyme Corporation. Fitness Chiropractic and Dr. Patel provide a therapy that is much more advanced and beneficial than any other I've experienced. He has healed injuries that plagued me for years. Through regular treatment and enzyme therapy he has allowed me to be pain free and make gains in my athletic career that I thought were no longer possible." - Craig Smith, Top 10 Professional Highland Games Athlete in the USA

Re: he's about to let the cat out of the bag!

"We have been getting some amazing results with the enzymes that one of my pro athletes has been using. He has not been able to throw for over a year now and is doing better than ever! He has broken three of his personal records and the forums have taken note. There is a lot of buzz about his most recent performance. His bruises are recovering much

quicker than before. He threw this past weekend and his hip felt better. His results are outstanding! He is really a believer now in the enzymes! He is about to let the cat out of the bag at nationals next week! Thank you for everything. We are going to be doing a lot of business together!"
- Sachin B. P. H B. K, A, DC.

SERIOUS ATHLETES...HERE IS YOUR PROOF!

I owned an enzyme company for many years called Transformation Enzyme Corporation. I bring this up because of the studies we did with Baylor University on our proteases. Since this is their research and they own it, I need to reveal my association. You can call and get the actual study from them if you like. It is too much to add to the weight of this book, but I will give you the highlights.

BACKGROUND:

Biochemically, physiologically, or clinically, inflammation can be defined as the biological reparation response following any disruption of the cell's structural or functional integrity by injurious agent(s) (internal or external) to the body. Based on this definition, injury brought about by sports or athletic activities will trigger a biological reparation response. Any therapeutic agent or dietary supplement that could enhance this biological reparation response would not only be helpful in athletic events but also in healthcare, as inflammation remains a common denominator to any health challenge. Transformation Enzyme Corporation (TEC) has formulated unique protease blends that provide numerous health benefits, most notably enhanced blood rheology, enhanced digestion of proteins, control of inflammation, and removal of protein debris from the circulatory system. These protease blends are comprised of several proteolytic enzymes that are able to sustain the acidic environment of the stomach without the addition of any excipients or coating agents. In an effort to specifically determine some of the biochemical actions of TEC's proteases on inflammation, a randomized, double-blinded, and placebo-controlled study was conducted at Baylor University under the direction of Dr. Darryn Willoughby.

OBJECTIVES:

The study was designed to determine the effects of TEC's proteolytic enzyme blend on muscle function and inflammation following strenuous exercise.

METHODS:

The study was conducted in a randomized, double-blinded, placebo-controlled manner. The subjects selected were 29 physically active, healthy males with the study guidelines by the Baylor University Institutional Review Board for Human Subjects. Following the baseline testing (T1), the participants (approximate average age of 22 and by consent and upon approval) were divided into two groups: one group of 14 received TEC's protease blend, whereas the other group of 15 received a placebo made up of cellulose. The participants took their respective supplements for 21 days. On day 21, the participants were subjected to another series of tests (T2), followed by an intense physical exercise regimen. Immediately following exercise, the tests were performed again (Post) as well as at 3, 24, and 48 hours. The participants continued taking the supplement until all testing had been completed.

RESULTS:

Transformation's protease blend proved to be more effective than the placebo in modulating several key inflammatory mediators and improving muscle strength as evidenced by the following data.

CONCLUSION:

Relative to the inflammatory mediators TNFa, IL1B, IL6, and IL12, the study results show that Transformation's protease blend has considerable potential for use in controlling inflammatory conditions in the body. The data also showed a beneficial decrease in COX2 activity, which shows these proteases can be used to manage pain without negative side effects. And according to the study results, the force production measurements showed protease supplementation led to improved muscle performance and an increase in muscle strength. The data provides scientific evidence confirming Transformation's consistently positive clinical results using proteolytic enzymes in the treatment of various health challenges characterized by inflammation.

DISCUSSION:

It is a known fact that inflammation is a common denominator in any pathological condition and occurs as long as the body is functioning. The causative agents may be varied, but the body's basic response is the same. While the Baylor study used strenuous exercise to induce inflammation, the data points are characteristic of any condition that causes cellular injury, such as trauma, infection, or tumor growth, for example.

Furthermore, studies have shown that decreases in IL12 help control some autoimmune disorders, suggesting TEC's protease as a good candidate in the management of certain degenerative disorders. Consequentially, the beneficial effect of protease on various inflammatory mediators, pain, and muscle strength could be extended to many other health challenges and implemented in a multitude of healthcare practices.

A controlled secretion of TNFa helps pro-inflammatory cytokines IL1 and IL6 respond appropriately, helping to modulate acute inflammation and control chronic inflammation. Modulated inflammation also reduces COX2 levels, which can result in less pain. This combination of decreased inflammation and lessened pain has the potential to enhance muscle performance, evidenced here as improved tolerance in sustaining the greater force production exercise load.

RECOMMENDATIONS:

Transformation's protease blend is recommended for acute and chronic inflammatory conditions that may arise from trauma, infection, or any degenerative disease process. These results also deserve special attention in the area of athletic performance, where protease would be a healthy alternative for supporting pain management, reduced recovery time, and enhanced muscle performance.

An objective of any wellness plan is to control inflammation either directly or indirectly. One of the functions of orally administered proteolytic enzymes as adjunct therapeutic agents is to trigger the inflammatory response and then also control it. Transformation's protease blend is a proven product for controlling inflammation, a valuable dietary supplement to be used as an adjunct therapeutic agent for the management of pain and to help control the debilitating effects of inflammation.

REFERENCES:

"Dietary Protease Supplementation Attenuates Eccentric Exercise Induced Force Production Decrements by Augmenting Leukocyte Activity and Systemic Inflammation." Thomas W. Buford, Matthew B. Cooke, Liz Redd, Geoffrey M. Hudson, Brian D. Shelmadine, Cecelia Curts, and Darryn S. Willoughby, Exercise and Biochemical Nutrition Laboratory, Baylor University, Waco, TX.

Chapter 18

Enzyme Labeling

There are now regulations governing potency in the labeling of enzymes, which can make it difficult to decide which enzyme product best meets your needs. To add to the confusion not everyone is following the rules. The accepted standard of labeling from the U.S. Food and Drug Administration is the Food Chemical Codex (FCC). Products labeled using the FCC will have unit measurements expressed as follows:

We are used to comparing food products based on weight, but with enzymes, it is the activity and potency, which we should be looking at. Be cautious of products which include fillers, or list contents by weight without listing proven activity units. You can call the company and ask for the units of activity and they should give them to you.

NOTE: You will see the word hydrolysis describing the chemical process in which a molecule of water is added to a substance to cause splitting or breaking down. Enzymes require water to do their job of digestion.

NOTE: The pH range in which these enzymes work is extremely important to digestion. They peak or are most available in their mid-range.

Enzyme Function	Enzyme Name	Source	pH Range	Notes
Hydrolysis of peptides and amino acids	Bromelain	*Ananas comosus* (pineapple stem)	4.0 - 9.0	Works in the small intestine & then blood for inflammation
	Papain	*Carica papaya* (green papaya fruit)	3.0 - 10.5	Best used topically on wounds
Inflammation, immune modulation, proteins	Peptidase	*Aspergillus oryzae*	3.25 - 7.5	Finishes the breaking down of proteases not completely digested in the stomach

Blood circulation & toxicity	Protease 3.0	*Aspergillus niger*	2.75 - 4.7	Works in stomach & throughout the digestive tract
Inflammation later in the digestive tract, into the liver, sinusitis	Protease 4.5	*Aspergillus oryzae var*	2.75 - 6.25	Same as the other proteases 3.0 but more towards alkaline
Edema, carry away toxicity, reduce pain, varicose veins	Protease 6.0	*Aspergillus oryzae*	2.75 - 7.0	Systemic protease, works in the blood
Hydrolysis of triglycerides	Lipase AN	*Aspergillus niger*	3.0 - 8.0	Tries to maintain pancreas as body ages so it can continue to produce lipase
Dietary fats & oil	Lipase	Gastric enzymes	3.0 - 8.0	Within the stomach to break down fatty acids
	Lipase	Liver enzymes	3.0 - 8.0	Carried by lymphatic system to liver
Starch, breads, pasta	Amylase	*Aspergillus oryzae*	3.0 - 7.0	Works with other enzymes to break down starch to sugar and other same carbohydrates
Digestion of polysaccharides, beans and vegetables	Alpha-galactosidase	*Aspergillus niger var*	2.5 - 7.5	Foods like greens or beans which are difficult to digest cause gas, but these enzymes help with their further breakdown
Sugars & desserts	Invertase	*Saccharomycs cerevisiae*	3.5 - 5.5	Breaks down the connection between glucose and fructose
Dairy sugars	Lactase	*Aspergillus oryzae*	3.0 - 8.0	Assists in the digestion of dairy products. Releases nutrients in dairy
Grains, rice	Beta-glucanase	*Trichoderma longibrachiatum*	2.0 - 7.0	Breaks down the glucans in wheat, barley and rye
Fiber	Macerase	*A. niger & T. longibrachiatum*	2.0 - 5.0	A complex enzyme to break down fibers in fruits

Cereals	Glucoamylase	*Aspergillus niger*	4.0 - 6.0	A different type of amylase helps break down starch foods, but also rids the body of dead white blood cells
Digestion of carbs	Diastase	*Hordeum vulgare* (barley malt)	4.0 - 9.0	Breaks down both sugar and starch in grains
	Xylanase	*Trichoderma longibrachiatum*	2.0 - 7.0	Naturally produced in the body by good microorganisms to break down fiber
Digestion of fiber, fruits, vegetables	Cellulase	*Trichoderma longibrachiatum*	2.0 - 8.0	Humans do not make this but when eating man-made fibers or plant cells, this enzyme is needed
And grains	Hemicellulase	*Aspergillus Niger*	3.0 - 5.5	Assist cellulase to break down bio-film
Skin on fruit	Pectinase	*Aspergillus Niger*	2.0 - 5.0	Plant cell walls
	Phytase	*Aspergillus Niger*	2.0 - 7.0	Liberates minerals from grains and helps in bone health

Appendix I

ABCs of Health

A. **Amino Acids** - Eat some protein at each meal to provide your body with the required amino acids. If it is difficult to eat enough healthy protein, or you are a vegetarian, drink protein drinks 1 to 2 times a day. The protein needs to be organic whey powder at 20 to 25 grams a scoop. Take supplemental digestive enzymes or supplemental protease enzymes with the drink to properly break down the protein powder into correct amino acids.

B. **Bacteria Ecology** - Our gastrointestinal tract contains an immensely complex ecology of bacteria. A typical adult harbors more than 500 different species of bacteria, representing dozens of different lifestyles and capabilities. The composition and distribution of this active colony varies with age, state of health, and diet. In contrast to the stomach and small intestine, the large intestine (colon) literally teems with bacteria. Take a healthy blend of probiotic at bedtime to promote a healthy ecology.

C. **Change** - If you have been diagnosed with a condition, one of the easiest things is to "change" what you are doing because what you are doing is not working for you. Think about what you can do to change your stressors. Change the way you think and eat. Maybe it is simply making sure you drink water and not soda drinks. Find your biochemical type and follow the suggestions—whatever...just change.

D. **Digestion** Take supplemental plant based digestive enzymes when eating to properly digest your food. Many things from stress to your age may now hinder your digestive processes.

E. **Enzymes** - Supplemental digestive and systemic enzymes can make a big difference as to how you feel or heal. Take the digestive enzymes with food or anytime you are feeling bloated. Add protease enzymes between meals or first thing in the AM and last in the PM to clean up the system and control inflammation.

F. **Food** - Pay attention to what you put in your mouth. Eat organic foods. These contain no genetically modified organisms (GMO), which are unrecognized proteins detrimental for your digestive tract. GMO foods lead to allergies in your digestive tract affecting your immune system. Eighty percent of your immune system lives in your digestive tract.

G. **GMO foods** - Give up these genetically modified foods containing animal, insect, virus, and bacteria proteins that our digestive system cannot recognize. This is where the gluten problems started. If you have gluten sensitivities, don't eat foods made with genetically-fed wheat, barley, or rye; and/or take supplemental enzymes with DPP-IV when you eat out or are not sure if the food you're eating has GMOs.

H. **Happiness** can directly produce good effects on your health. Research has shown that happy people have a higher level of Immunoglobin A, an important immune system protein. Immunoglobin A helps your body protect itself from respiratory disease. Happiness also helps block harmful hormones from getting released in your body. It's even been scientifically shown that happiness can alter your DNA! A team of researchers at UCLA showed that people with a deep sense of happiness had lower levels of inflammatory gene expression and stronger antiviral and antibody responses.

I. **Imagine** good things and balanced health for your body. Imagination makes you more knowledgeable and interested in moving forward with your life.

J. **Joy** - A great feeling of pleasure—the joy of being alive. Surround yourself with joyful people.

K. **Kindness** - As the saying goes, "Try a little kindness." It is a virtue we can learn to develop.

L. **Love** represents many feelings, thoughts, and attitudes. The healthiest love we can have is for "self" because you are of a higher power.

M. **Meditation** is a practice in which we train our minds to realize a benefit or technique to enjoy an indestructible sense of well-being while engaging in life. Meditation is often used to clear the mind and ease many health issues, such as high blood pressure, depression, and anxiety.

N. **Nap** if possible—it will make you feel better. Napping was found to be both physiologically and psychologically beneficial. Napping for 20 minutes can help refresh the mind, improve overall alertness, boost mood, and increase productivity.

O. **Organic food** is important to add to your diet, and when possible, eat totally organic and/or buy from your local food co-op. These foods do not contain genetically modified insects, bacteria, and virus or animal proteins. Eat grass-fed beef, organic eggs, and wild fish.

P. **Proteins** - Eat enough healthy proteins to feed your body, maintain good health, and provide the strength to fight back against disease.

Q. **Quality of life** is the perceived value of daily life and well-being we are enjoying.

R. **Read** to educate yourself and discover the things you love most in life. If ill, educate yourself to make better choices about your health.

S. **Sleep** is extremely important in so many ways. Our organs begin their detoxification in the middle of the night. Not sleeping enough, and not sleeping well, is not OK. As a matter of fact, there is quite a price to pay. It may surprise you to learn that chronic sleep deprivation, for whatever reason, significantly affects your health, performance, safety, job, and quality of life.

T. **T cells** are your helper cells, which your immune system counts on. They are a type of lymphocyte (white blood cell), have memory from past infections, and are used to call on the killer cells for help to protect you. It is important to have healthy blood. Protease systemic enzymes assist in balancing your blood system.

U. **Unwell** - How does that refer to you? All your blood tests come out normal and every doctor you see treats something different until you realize no one knows how to treat "unwell"—it has to have a diagnostic name. They have now come up with one "catch all" name: NID or neuro-immune disease. NID refers to a group of illnesses that are the result of acquired dysregulation of both the immune system and the nervous system, often resulting in lifelong disease and disability. These diseases impact tens of millions of people around the world, yet those who suffer have no FDA-approved treatments for underlying causes of the diseases or methods to prevent others from becoming ill. If that sounds scary to you, do not let it. Follow the ABCs of Health and pull yourself out—I did.

V. **Value of exercise** - Without regular physical exercise, our bodies degenerate faster and our lifespans are shorter as well. It is a well-known fact that regular physical exercise not only strengthens our muscles, tendons, ligaments, bones, and internal organs, and it makes us more immune to various kinds of diseases. Apart from these benefits, it also makes us look leaner and younger and gives us a sense of well-being, happiness, and confidence.

W. **Water** is a requirement by every cell in your body, but the most important reason-it is necessary to our metabolic and supplemental enzymes. Enzymes, whether those we make in our bodies or those we take by mouth, require water to work. Our blood plasma needs water, as does every organ. Those that suggest no one drink water with meals do not understand biochemistry or enzymology.

X. **Example** - Become a fine example of a healthy human being that is living life to the fullest. Lead by example.

Y. **YHVH** is the spelling of the sacred name of GOD. The name came to be regarded as too sacred to be spoken, and the vowel sounds are uncertain. Have you wondered why we can think ourselves well or heal aspects of our mind by forgiveness or changing our belief?

We may discover that the answer to this question is precisely the key that lies at the heart of our most deeply held beliefs and traditions. Almost universally, ancient accounts tell us that with the first of our kind, our species was infused with what has been described as a special "spark," a mysterious thread of spiritual essence that eternally joins us with others of our kind and our Creator. It is this spark that sets us apart from all other forms of life. Perhaps it's the same force that imbues uniqueness into our genetic code as well.

We are not alone. We are here "on purpose," as the result of an intentional act of creation. We are inextricably linked to one another and all life. We share a unique trait—the essence of God—in a way that sets us apart from all other life on Earth.

Preserved within each cell of the estimated 6 billion inhabitants of our world, God's message is repeated, again and again, to form the building blocks of our existence. This ancient message from the day of our origins—the same message—remains within each of us today, regardless of race, color, beliefs, actions, lifestyle, religion, or heritage. The odds that this relationship has occurred by chance are approximately 1 in 200,000.

From the smallest single-celled organisms to the estimated 100 trillion cells that make up a single human body, the code of each life form is made from different arrangements of these four basic elements. These are Hydrogen, Nitrogen, Oxygen, and Carbon. The key to translating the code of our DNA into an ancient and meaningful language is to apply the discovery that converts elements to letters based upon their matching values.

An analysis of the number values representing the DNA in our human cells (YHVG) and the values that represent the name of God (YHVH) reveals that, even though we share in the attributes of God's name, we are not equal to God.

Hydrogen becomes the Hebrew letter Yod (Y),
Nitrogen becomes the letter Hey (H),
Oxygen becomes the letter Vav (V), and
Carbon becomes Gimel (G).

These substitutions now reveal that the ancient form of God's name, YH, exists as the literal chemistry of our genetic code. By replacing the elements of our DNA with their equivalents of Hebrew letters, we reveal the message that is spelled out within each cell of each of our bodies. As we change our perception, in a very literal sense, we redefine our bodies as well. The ability to improve immune functions; shift our hormone levels; and alter heart rate, breath, and metabolism simply by changing the way we feel is well-documented in the scientific and medical literature. To read more: *The God Code* by Greg Braden.

Z. **Zeal** – Living with zeal or passion for what you do in life gives you great energy. Gives you a reason to get up in the morning and pursue life with enthusiasm and energy.

Appendix II

Healthy Aging

1. Eat fresh organic foods.

2. Eat meats that are grass-fed, no hormones.

3. Drink adequate amount of pure water for your body and enzyme requirements.

4. Ingest Supplemental Digestive Enzymes with each meal.

5. Ingest Supplemental Protease (proteolytic) enzymes between meals such as first in AM, mid-afternoon, and last in PM before bed.

6. Take Supplemental Probiotic blends before bed if needing more large intestine balance. Take at both the AM and PM.

7. Ingest natural nutrients (void of synthetic vitamins), or drink natural green drinks.

8. Following exercise, take inflammatory repair enzymes. You will maintain muscle and skip the soreness.

9. Enjoy adequate sleep each night. Get in a habit of going to bed and awakening around the same time daily.

Increasing your knowledge of how the body works ***DEEPENS*** your understanding of health and how you can be better prepared to take care of yourself. Let's look at the word ***DEEPENS***. Each letter offers a key component that you will need for healthy aging.

D = Drink pure water

E = Eat real food—not GMO or packaged

E = Enzymes with each meal and/or between

P = Probiotics for internal harmony

E = Exercise with weights and walk

N = Natural nutrients—not synthetics

S = Sleep for repair

Scientific References

Ajslev TA, Andersen CS, Gamborg M, Sorensen TI, Jess T. Childhood overweight after establishment of the gut microbiota: the role of delivery mode, pre-pregnancy weight and early administration of antibiotics. Int. J. Obes. 2011;35:522-529.

Bäckhed F, et al. The gut microbiota as an environmental factor that regulates fat storage. Proc. Natl Acad. Sci. USA 2004;101,15718-15723.

Bouchard C, Tremblay A, Després JP, Nadeau A, Lupien PJ, Thériault G, Dussault J, Moorjani S, Pinault S, Fournier G. The response to long-term overfeeding in identical twins. N Engl J Med. 1990 May 24;322(21):1477-82.

Brown JC, Jiang X. Prevalence of antibiotic-resistant bacteria in herbal products. J Food Prot. 2008 Jul;71(7):1486-90.

Campos J, Mourão J, Pestana N, Peixe L, Novais C, Antunes P. Microbiological quality of ready-to-eat salads: an underestimated vehicle of bacteria and clinically relevant antibiotic resistance genes.Int J Food Microbiol. 2013 Sep 16;166(3):464-70.

Candela M, et al. Interaction of probiotic Lactobacillus and Bifidobacterium strains with human intestinal epithelial cells: adhesion properties, competition against enteropathogens and modulation of IL-8 production. Int. J. Food Microbiol. 2008;125:286-292.

Cani PD, Amar J, Iglesias MA, Poggi M, Knauf C, Bastelica D, et al. Metabolic endotoxemia initiates obesity and insulin resistance. Diabetes 2007;56:1761-1772.

Cani PD, Osto M, Geurts L, Everard A. Involvement of gut microbiota in the development of low-grade inflammation and type 2 diabetes associated with obesity. Gut Microbes. 2012 July 1;3(4):279-288.

Carvalho BM, Saad MJ. Influence of gut microbiota on subclinical inflammation and insulin resistance. Mediators Inflamm. 2013;986734.

Cho I, Yamanishi S, Cox L, Methe BA, Zavadil J, Li K, Gao Z, Mahana D, Raju K, Teitler I, et al. Antibiotics in early life alter the murine colonic microbiome and adiposity. Nature. 2012;488:621-626.

Claesson MJ, et al. Gut microbiota composition correlates with diet and health in the elderly. Nature 2012;488:178-184.

Cotillard A, et al. Dietary intervention impact on gut microbial gene richness. Nature 2013 Aug 29;500:585-588.

De Filippo C, et al. Impact of diet in shaping gut microbiota revealed by a comparative study in children from Europe and rural Africa. Proc. Natl Acad. Sci. USA 2010;107:14691-14696.

Dethlefsen L, Huse S, Sogin ML, Relman DA. The pervasive effects of an antibiotic on the human gut microbiota, as revealed by deep 16S rRNA sequencing. PLoS Biol. 2008;6:e280.

Dethlefsen L, Relman DA. Incomplete recovery and individualized responses of the human distal gut microbiota to repeated antibiotic perturbation. Proc Natl Acad Sci USA 2011;108(Suppl 1):4554-61.

Devillard E, McIntosh FM, Duncan SH, Wallace RJ. Metabolism of linoleic acid by human gut bacteria: different routes for biosynthesis of conjugated linoleic acid. J. Bacteriol. 2007;189:2566-2570.

Devillard E, McIntosh FM, Duncan SH, Wallace RJ. Metabolism of linoleic acid by human gut bacteria: different routes for biosynthesis of conjugated linoleic acid. J. Bacteriol. 2007;189:2566-2570.

Dicksved J, et al. Molecular analysis of the gut microbiota of identical twins with Crohn's disease. ISME J. 2008;2:716-727.

Duncan SH, et al. Reduced dietary intake of carbohydrates by obese subjects results in decreased concentrations of butyrate and butyrate-producing bacteria in feces. Appl. Environ. Microbiol. 2007;73:1073-1078.

Duran GM, Marshall DL. Ready-to-eat shrimp as an international vehicle of antibiotic-resistant bacteria. J Food Prot. 2005 Nov;68(11):2395-401.

Forsythe P, Kunze WA, Bienenstock J. On communication between gut microbes and the brain. Curr Opin Gastroenterol. 2012;28:557-562.

Fukuda S, et al. Bifidobacteria can protect from enteropathogenic infection through production of acetate. Nature 2011;469:543-547.

Goodman AL, Kallstrom G, Faith JJ, Reyes A, et al. Extensive personal human gut microbiota culture collections characterized and manipulated in gnotobiotic mice. Proceedings of the national Academy of Sciences of the United States of America. 2010;108:346-357.

Halden RU, Paull DH. Co-occurrence of triclocarban and triclosan in US water resources. Environ Sci Technol. 2005 Mar 15;39(6):1420-6.

Hara N, Alkanani AK, Ir D, et al. The role of the intestinal microbiota in type 1 diabetes. Clin Immunol. 2013;146:112-119.

Human Microbiome Project Consortium. Structure, function, and diversity of the healthy human microbiome. Nature 2012;486:207-214.

Jakobsson HE, et al. Short-term antibiotic treatment has differing long-term impacts on the human throat and gut microbiome. PLoS ONE 2010;5s:e9836.

Jalanka-Tuovinen J, Salonen A, Nikkilä J, et al. Intestinal microbiota in healthy adults: temporal analysis reveals individual and common core and relation to intestinal symptoms. PLoS One. 2011;6:e23035.

Jernberg C, Lofmark S, Edlund C, Jansson JK. Long-term ecological impacts of antibiotic administration on the human intestinal microbiota. ISME J. 2007;1:56-66.

Kallus SJ, Brandt LJ. The intestinal microbiota and obesity. J Clin Gastroenterol. 2012;46:16-24.

Le Chatelier E, et al. Richness of human gut microbiome correlates with metabolic markers.Nature. 2013 Aug 29;500(7464):541-6.

Lee YK, Menezes JS, Umesaki Y, Mazmanian SK. Proinflammatory T-cell responses to gut microbiota promote experimental autoimmune encephalomyelitis. Proc Natl Acad Sci USA. 2011;108(Suppl 1):4615-4622.

Lepage P, et al. Twin study indicates loss of interaction between microbiota and mucosa of patients with ulcerative colitis. Gastroenterology 2011;141:227-236.

Logan AC, Rao AV, Irani D. Chronic fatigue syndrome: lactic acid bacteria may be of therapeutic value. Medical hypotheses 2003;60(6):915-923.

Lozupone CA, Stombaugh JI, Gordon JI, Jansson JK, Knight R. Diversity, stability and resilience of the human gut microbiota. Nature 2012 Sep 13;489(7415):220-30.

Luecke RW, McMillen WN, Thorp F. The effect of vitamin B12, animal protein factor and streptomycin on the growth of young pigs. Arch Biochem 1950;26:326-7.

Lupton JR. Microbial degradation products influence colon cancer risk: the butyrate controversy. J. Nutr. 2004;134;479-482.

Manichanh C, et al. Reduced diversity of faecal microbiota in Crohn's disease revealed by a metagenomic approach. Gut 2006;55:205-211.

Moore PR, Evenson A, Luckey TD, McCoy E, Elvejem CA, Hart EB. Use of sulfasuxidine, streptothricin, and streptomycin in nutritional studies with the chick. J Biol Chem 1946;165(2):437-41.

Murphy EF, Cotter PD, Hogan A, et al. Divergent metabolic outcomes arising from targeted manipulation of the gut microbiota in diet-induced obesity. Gut. 2013;62:220-226.

Olszak T, et al. Microbial exposure during early life has persistent effects on natural killer T cell function. Science 2012;336:489-493.

Opal SM. Endotoxins and other sepsis triggers. Contrib Nephrol. 2010;167:14-24.

Parnell JA, Reimer RA Weight loss during oligofructose supplementation is associated with decreased ghrelin and increased peptide YY in overweight and obese adults. Am J Clin Nutr 2009;89:1751-9.

Pontzer H, Raichlen DA, Wood BM, Mabulla AZ, Racette SB, Marlowe FW. Hunter-gatherer energetics and human obesity. PLoS One. 2012;7(7):e40503.

Prentice AM, Black AE, Coward WA, Cole TJ. Energy expenditure in overweight and obese adults in affluent societies: an analysis of 319 doubly-labelled water measurements. Eur J Clin Nutr. 1996 Feb;50(2):93-7.

Qin J, et al. A human gut microbial gene catalogue established by metagenomic sequencing. Nature 2010;464:59-65.

Ramachanrappa S, Farooqi IS. Genetics approaches to understanding human obesity. Journal of Clinical investigation. 2011;121:2080-2086.

Rossi M, Amaretti A, Raimondi S. Folate production by probiotic bacteria. Nutrients. 2011 Jan;3(1):118-34.

Scher JU, Sczesnak A, Longman RS, et al. Expansion of intestinal Prevotella copri correlates with enhanced susceptibility to arthritis. eLife. 2013;2:e01202.

Swinburn BA, Sacks G, Lo SK, Westerterp KR, Rush EC, Rosenbaum M, Luke A, Schoeller DA, DeLany JP, Butte NF, Ravussin E. Estimating the changes in energy flux that characterize the rise in obesity prevalence. Am J Clin Nutr. 2009 Jun;89(6):1723-8.

Tang WH, Wang Z, Levison BS, et al. Intestinal microbial metabolism of phosphatidylcholine and cardiovascular risk. N Engl J Med. 2013;368:1575-1584.

Ternak G. Antibiotics may act as growth/obesity promoters in humans as an inadvertent result of antibiotic pollution. Med Hypotheses 2005.

Thuny F, Richet H, Casalta JP, Angelakis E, Habib G, Raoult D. Vancomycin treatment of infective endocarditis is linked with recently acquired obesity. PLoS One 2010;5(2):e9074.10.1371/journal.pone.0009074

Trasande L, Blustein J, Liu M, Corwin E, Cox LM, Blaser MJ. Infant antibiotic exposures and early-life body mass. Int J Obes (Lond). 2013 Jan;37(1):16-23.

Tremblay A, Despres JP, Therault G, Fournier G, Bouchard C. Overfeeding and energy expenditure in humans. Am J Clin Nutr 1993:56:857-62.

Turnbaugh PJ, et al. An obesity-associated gut microbiome with increased capacity for energy harvest. Nature 2006;444:1027-1031.

Turnbaugh PJ, et al. An obesity-associated gut microbiome with increased capacity for energy harvest. Nature 2006;444:1027–1031.

Vaarala O, Atkinson MA, Neu J. The "perfect storm" for type 1 diabetes: the complex interplay between intestinal microbiota, gut permeability, and mucosal immunity. Diabetes. 2008;57:2555-2562.

Wang Y, Kasper LH. The role of microbiome in central nervous system disorders. Brain Behav Immun. 2013 Dec 25.

Wu GD, Chen J, Hoffmann C, Bittinger K, Chen YY, Keilbaugh SA, Bewtra M, Knights D, Walters WA, Knight R, Sinha R, Gilroy E, Gupta K, Baldassano R, Nessel L, Li H, Bushman FD, Lewis JD. Linking long-term dietary patterns with gut microbial enterotypes. Science. 2011 Oct 7;334(6052):105-8.

Xiao S, Zhao L. Gut microbiota-based translational biomarkers to prevent metabolic syndrome via nutritional modulation. FEMS Microbiol Ecol. 2013 Nov 12.

Yatsunenko T, et al. Human gut microbiome viewed across age and geography. Nature 2012;486:222–227.

About the Author

Dr. DicQie Fuller-Looney holds a Ph.D. in Nutrition and Health Sciences with more than three decades of clinical experience specializing in enzyme therapy and nutrition. Her emphasis includes a special interest in patterns of inherited traits, biochemical individualism, digestion, blood rheology, and diet, combining nutrition and enzyme therapy supported by various validation systems. Research and clinical results are obtained to emphasize the importance of enzyme therapy in nutrition and disease.

Dr. Fuller-Looney's interest in holistic health began over 40 years ago when her daughter, Coleen, became ill and was given a short time to live. Frustrated with traditional treatments, she began to research natural and non-traditional therapies for an answer. Through extensive research and data, Dr. Fuller-Looney was able to monitor everything her daughter consumed (vitamins, minerals, food, etc.). Soon she discovered her daughter's inability to properly digest, utilize, and eliminate food. With this new knowledge, her research turned to Dr. Edward Howell's work on plant enzymes. Coleen began the plant enzyme supplementation and experienced rapid and lasting results. From that point on, Dr. Fuller-Looney began to use plant enzyme supplementation clinically and personally, and not only is her daughter alive and well, but enzyme therapy has become Dr. Fuller-Looney's life's work.

As a leading spokesperson for enzymes, Dr. Fuller-Looney is continually sought after for health seminars, conventions, and committee meetings. She has appeared on ABC, PBS, and several national radio talk shows. Her significant contributions to the rapidly growing awareness of the importance of enzymes and nutrition have been honored in Who's Who of Women Executives, Who's Who of American Women, and Woman of the Year 1990.

Dr. Fuller-Looney has published extensively, including articles on the use of enzymes in nutrition, body typing, glandular therapy, and appetite and weight control. In addition to *The Healing Power of Enzymes*, she has co-authored *Living Longer: Questions You Never Knew To Ask, Answers You Can't Live Without* with Dick Couey, Ph.D., of Baylor University and *The M Club: Survive Menopause and Feel Great Again with the Healing Power of Enzymes*.